3738

cancelled
9/9/05

# Recent developments
# in orthopaedic surgery

# SIR  HARRY  PLATT

## Bt., M.D., M.S., LL.D., F.R.C.S., F.A.C.S.

### 1886 - 1986

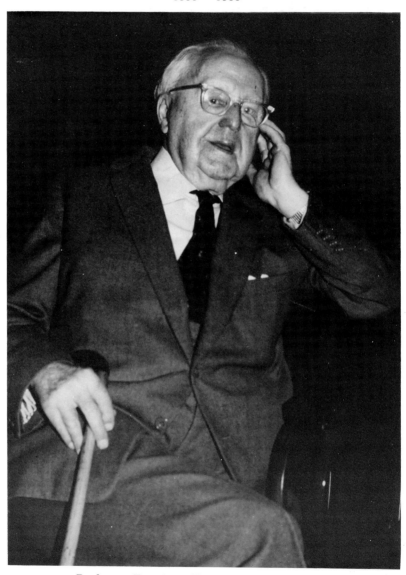

Professor Emeritus, University of Manchester
Past President, Royal College of Surgeons of England
Past President, SICOT

# Recent developments in orthopaedic surgery

*Editors*

# J. Noble, C. S. B. Galasko

**Manchester University Press**

Published by
Manchester University Press
Oxford Road, Manchester M13 9PL, UK

and

27 South Main Street, Wolfeboro, New Hampshire 03894-2069, USA


British Library cataloguing in publication data

Recent developments in orthopaedic surgery.
   1. Orthopaedic surgery
   I. Noble, J.   II. Galasko, C.S.B.
   616'.3     RD731



Library of Congress cataloging   in publication data applied for




ISBN 0-7190-2542-7 cased

Printed and bound in Great Britain
by Biddles Ltd, Guildford and King's Lynn

# CONTENTS

# CONTENTS

# PREFACE

In October 1986, Surgeons from around the World gathered in Manchester to honour the doyen of orthopaedic surgery, Sir Harry Platt, on his one hundredth birthday. In this book are published the papers chosen for presentation at the Meeting. Orthopaedic surgery is a rapidly developing subject in which many advances have occurred during the past few years. It is an enormous specialty with many advancing fronts and it is not possible to consider all the recent developments in orthopaedic surgery in a book of this size; rather those branches of orthopaedic surgery, in which Sir Harry Platt was particularly interested, were chosen.

The book is mainly devoted to developments in shoulder surgery; advances in the treatment of bone tumours, both primary and metastatic; recent developments in children's orthopaedic surgery; the management of complicated fractures and nerve injuries; spinal surgery; the surgical treatment of arthritis; and new developments in imaging techniques. Potential developments in orthopaedic surgery are also described. The book is aimed at those Orthopaedic Surgeons and trainees who wish to keep abreast of recent developments in orthopaedic surgery.

The Editors hope that the book will also serve as an everlasting memory to one of the greatest Orthopaedic Surgeons of all time, Sir Harry Platt, who made so many contributions to the development of our specialty.

C.S.B.G.

J.N.

(Manchester, 1987).

# ACKNOWLEDGEMENTS

We are very grateful to the following, without whom this Festschrift would not have been possible:

Mrs. Janice Farrell for all her skilled secretarial help, and in particular for typing all the manuscripts.

Miss Stella Rushton and Dr. Carol Evans for checking all the References.

The members of the Department of Orthopaedic Surgery, University of Manchester, who made the Meeting possible.

The contributors to the book, particularly for submitting their articles within the deadline and for allowing the editors to reduce the size of their contributions to the limits agreed with the publishers.

# LIST OF CONTRIBUTORS

**Mohamed Arafa** FRCS, FRCSEd(Orth)
Lecturer in Orthopaedic Surgery, University of Manchester, U.K.
**Massimo Baratelli** MD
Assistant, Orthopaedic Research Unit, Istituto di Patologia e Clinica dell' Apparato Locomotore, Milan, Italy.
**James E. Bateman** MD, FRCS(C)
Surgeon-in-Chief (Emeritus), Orthopaedic and Arthritic Hospital, Toronto.
Associate Professor of Surgery, University of Toronto, Canada.
**Peter Beighton** MD, PhD, FRCP, DCH
Professor of Human Genetics, University of Cape Town.
Director of MRC Research Unit for Inherited Skeletal Disorders, South Africa.
**F. Howard Beddow** MChOrth, FRCSEd
Consultant Orthopaedic Surgeon, Royal Liverpool Hospital.
Part-time Clinical Lecturer in Orthopaedic Surgery, University of Liverpool, U.K.
**J. A. Betts** FRCS
Consultant Orthopaedic Surgeon, Queen Elizabeth Hospital, Gateshead.
Honorary Lecturer, Department of Orthopaedics, University of Newcastle-on-Tyne, U.K.
**David E. Beverland** MD, FRCS
Senior Orthopaedic Registrar, Musgrave Park Hospital, Belfast, U.K.
**Benjamin E. Bierbaum** MD
Orthopaedic Surgeon-in-Chief, New England Baptist Hospital, Boston.
Clinical Professor of Orthopaedic Surgery, Tufts University School of Medicine, Boston, U.S.A.
**Rolfe Birch** FRCS
Consultant Orthopaedic Surgeon, St. Mary's Hospital, London,
and the Royal National Orthopaedic Hospital, Stanmore, Middlesex, U.K.

**G. Blatter** MD

Oberarzt, Department of Orthopedics, Kantonsspital, St. Gallen, Switzerland.

**Noel J. Blockey** FRCSEng, FRCS Glas, MChOrth

Consultant Orthopaedic Surgeon, Royal Hospital for Sick Children and Western Infirmary, Glasgow.

Barclay Lecturer in Orthopaedics, University of Glasgow, U.K.

**Stephen P. Bogosian** MD

Otto E. Aufranc Fellow, New England Baptist Hospital.

Clinical Instructor, Tufts University School of Medicine, Boston, Massachusetts, U.S.A.

**Murray Brookes** MA, DM, DLO

Professor of Orthopaedic Anatomy, United Medical and Dental Schools, Guy's Hospital, London, U.K.

**Paul D. Byers** BSc, MDCM, DCP, PhD, FRCPath

Head, Department of Morbid Anatomy, and Honorary Consultant, Institute of Orthopaedics, London.

Reader, University of London, U.K.

**Ruggero Cadossi** MD

Assistant Professor of Internal Medicine, University of Modena, Italy.

**James M. Carey** MD

Director of Orthopaedic Education, Newington Children's Hospital, Connecticut, U.S.A.

**D. B. Case** MChOrth, FRCS

Senior Consultant Orthopaedic Surgeon, Royal Preston Hospital, Preston, U.K.

**C. L. Colton** FRCS, FRCSEd(Orth)

Consultant in Orthopaedic and Trauma Surgery, University Hospital, Queen's Medical Centre, Nottingham, U.K.

**T. Derek V. Cooke** MA, FRCS(C)

Professor of Surgery, Division of Orthopaedics.

Chairman of the Clinical Mechanics Group, Queen's University, Kingston, Ontario.

Attending Staff, Kingston General Hospital; Consultant, Hotel Dieu and St. Mary's of the Lake Hospitals, Kingston, Ontario, Canada.

**John Dove** FRCS

Consultant Orthopaedic Surgeon, Hartshill Orthopaedic Hospital, Stoke-on-Trent, U.K.

**Khalid J. Drabu** FRCS
Orthopaedic Senior Registrar, Hope Hospital, Salford, U.K.

**Gwyn A. Evans** FRCS, FRCS(Orth)
Consultant and Director of Children's Orthopaedics, Orthopaedic Hospital, Oswestry, U.K.

**Malcolm W. Fidler** MS, FRCS
Orthopaedic Surgeon, Onze Lieve Vrouwe Gasthuis, Amsterdam.
Consultant Orthopaedic Surgeon, Netherlands Cancer Institute, Amsterdam, Holland.

**Bryn Fisher** RN
Clinical Research Assistant, Queen's University, Kingston, Ontario, Canada.

**David J. Ford** FRCS, FRCSEd(Orth)
Registrar in Orthopaedics, Robert Jones and Agnes Hunt Orthopaedic Hospital, Oswestry, U.K.

**P. L. Frank** FRCSEd
Consultant Orthopaedic Surgeon, Hope Hospital, Salford.
Honorary Associate Lecturer, Department of Orthopaedic Surgery, University of Manchester, U.K.

**Ian S. Fyfe** FRCSEd, FRCSEng, FRCSEd(Orth)
Consultant Orthopaedic Surgeon, Northwick Park Hospital, Harrow, Middlesex, U.K.

**James R. Gage** MD
Director of Orthopaedic Research, Newington Children's Hospital, Connecticut, U.S.A.

**Charles S. B. Galasko** MSc, ChM, FRCSEng, FRCSEd
Professor of Orthopaedic Surgery, University of Manchester.
Honorary Consultant Orthopaedic Surgeon, Hope Hospital and Royal Manchester Children's Hospital, Salford, U.K.

**Mats Hamberg** MD
Department of Orthopaedic Surgery, University Hospital, Uppsala, Sweden.

**Tetsuya Hara** MD, DrMedSci
Head of Department of Orthopaedic Surgery, Tokyo Municipal Hiroo Hospital.
Lecturer, Department of Orthopaedic Surgery, University of Tokyo, Japan.

**Kevin Hardinge** MChOrth, FRCS
Consultant Orthopaedic Surgeon, Wrightington Hospital, Lancashire.
Honorary Associate Lecturer, Department of Orthopaedic Surgery,

University of Manchester, U.K.

**J. G. Hardy** PhD

Senior Medical Physicist, Medical Physics Department, University Hospital, Queen's Medical Centre, Nottingham, U.K.

**David M. Heilbronner** MD

Assistant Professor of Orthopaedics and Rehabilitation,

Assistant Professor of Paediatrics, University of Virginia School of Medicine, Charlottesville, Virginia, U.S.A.

**John P. Hodgkinson** FRCS

Orthopaedic Senior Registrar, Royal Preston Hospital, Preston, U.K.

**John D. Hsu** MD, CM, FACS

Clinical Professor, Department of Orthopaedics, University of Southern California School of Medicine.

Attending Orthopaedic Surgeon, Rancho Los Amigos Medical Center, Downey, California, U.S.A.

**Angus William Hughes** FRCS

Lecturer in Orthopaedic Surgery, University of Glasgow, U.K.

**Malcolm I. V. Jayson** MD, MSc, FRCP

Professor of Rheumatology, University of Manchester Rheumatic Diseases Centre, Hope Hospital, Salford, U.K.

**M. R. K. Karpinski** MChOrth, FRCSEd(Orth)

Senior Orthopaedic Registrar, Harlow Wood Orthopaedic Hospital, Nottinghamshire, U.K.

**W. George Kernohan** PhD

Lecturer, Queen's University of Belfast, Musgrave Park Hospital, Belfast, U.K.

**John R. Kirkup** FRCS, DHM

Consultant Orthopaedic Surgeon, Bath and Wessex Orthopaedic Hospital. Archivist, British Orthopaedic Association, U.K.

**P. S. London** MBE, FRCS, MFOM, FACEM(Hon)

Senior Surgeon, Birmingham Accident Hospital.

Senior Clinical Tutor, University of Birmingham, U.K.

**Saverio Lori** MD

Resident in Orthopaedic Surgery, Second University of Rome, Italy.

**Gerald F. McCoy** MD, FRCS

Orthopaedic Senior Registrar, Musgrave Park Hospital, Belfast, U.K.

**Allan M. McKelvie** MS, FACS

Orthopaedic Surgeon, Washington D.C., U.S.A.

**S. J. McLoughlin** FRCS

Orthopaedic Registrar, North Manchester Hospitals, U.K.

**Edward B. MacMahon** MD, FACS

Assistant Professor, Georgetown University Hospital, Washington.

Consultant Orthopaedic Surgeon, VA Medical Center, Washington, U.S.A.

**Loredana Mastidoro** MD

Intern, Orthopaedic Department, Second University of Rome, Italy.

**R. J. Minns** BEng, MSc, PhD

Senior Physicist, Regional Medical Physics Department, Durham Unit, Dryburn Hospital, Durham.

Visiting Research Fellow, Department of Engineering, University of Durham, U.K.

**Raymond A. B. Mollan** MD, FRCS, FRCSI

Professor of Orthopaedic Surgery, The Queen's University of Belfast.

Honorary Consultant Orthopaedic Surgeon, Musgrave Park Hospital, Belfast, U.K.

**Alessandro Dal Monte** MD

Professor of Orthopaedic Surgery, University of Bologna.

Chief of Orthopaedic Service, Istituto Ortopedico Rizzoli, Bologna, Italy.

**Maurizio Monteleone** MD

Professor of Orthopaedic Surgery, University of Rome.

Head Surgeon, First University of Rome.

Head Surgeon and Director of Orthopaedic Department, Second University of Rome, Italy.

**Peter Morris** FFARCS, DCH

Consultant Anaesthetist, Royal Manchester Children's Hospital.

Honorary Associate Lecturer, Departments of Anaesthesia and Child Health, University of Manchester.

Visiting Honorary Professor, Department of Aeronautical and Mechanical Engineering, University of Salford, U.K.

**D. S. Muckle** MD, FRCS

Consultant Orthopaedic Surgeon, Middlesborough General Hospital, Middlesborough.

Visiting Research Fellow, Department of Engineering, University of Durham, U.K.

**R. C. Mulholland** FRCS

Consultant Orthopaedic Surgeon, University Hospital, Nottingham.

Consultant Orthopaedic Surgeon, Harlow Wood Orthopaedic Hospital, Nottinghamshire, U.K.

**Akira Nagano** MD, DrMedSci
Associate Professor, Department of Orthopaedic Surgery, University of Tokyo, Japan.

**Geoffrey F. Newton** FRCSEng
Consultant Orthopaedic Surgeon, Bretby Hall Orthopaedic Hospital, Bretby, Staffordshire and Derbyshire Royal Infirmary Hospital, Derby, U.K

**Jonathan Noble** ChM, FRCSEd
Consultant Orthopaedic Surgeon, Hope Hospital, Salford.
Honorary Associate Lecturer, Department of Orthopaedic Surgery, University of Manchester, U.K.

**Gisèle Novakovitch** MD
Chief of Service, Department of Cryobiology, Centre de Transfusion Sanquine, Marseille, France.

**John P. O'Brien** PhD, FRCSEd, FACS
Consultant Surgeon in Spinal Disorders.
Honorary Lecturer in Spinal Surgery, Department of Neurosurgery, The London Hospital, London, U.K.

**Sven Olerud** MD
Professor of Orthopaedic Surgery, University Hospital, Uppsala, Sweden.

**Robert Owen** MChOrth, FRCS
Professor of Orthopaedic Surgery, University of Liverpool, U.K.

**Matteo Parrini** MD
Resident, Orthopaedic Research Unit, Istituto di Patologia e Clinica dell'Apparato Locomotore, Milan, Italy.

**D. G. Poitout** MD
Professor of Orthopaedic Surgery and Chief of Service, Hospital Nord, Universite d'Aix, Marseille, France.

**Gabriele Poli** MD
Assistant, Department of Orthopaedic Surgery, Istituto Ortopedico Rizzoli, Bologna, Italy.

**Hamish Potts** FRCSEd
Orthopaedic Registrar, Hope Hospital and Royal Manchester Children's Hospital, Salford, U.K.

**Laurence Read** BSc, FRCS
Consultant Orthopaedic Surgeon, Bromsgrove and Redditch District General

Hospital, Redditch, U.K.

**Thomas R. Redfern** MChOrth, FRCSEd
Orthopaedic Senior Registrar, Royal Liverpool Hospital and University of Liverpool, U.K.

**Fabrizio Remotti** MD
Resident in Orthopaedic Surgery, Second University of Rome, Italy.

**Clare M. Rimnac** PhD
Assistant Scientist and Assistant Professor of Applied Biomechanics (Surgery), The Hospital for Special Surgery and Cornell University Medical College, New York, U.S.A.

**P. A. Ring** MS, FRCSEng
Consultant Orthopaedic Surgeon, East Surrey Hospital, and Joint Replacement Unit, Dorking Hospital, Surrey, U.K.

**E. Raymond S. Ross** FRCSEd, FRACS
Consultant Orthopaedic Surgeon, Wythenshawe Hospital, Manchester. Honorary Associate Lecturer, University of Manchester, U.K.

**Carter R. Rowe** MD, DSc
Associate Clinical Professor (Emeritus), Harvard Medical School, Boston. Senior Orthopaedic Surgeon, Massachusetts General Hospital, Boston, U.S.A.

**Bahman Sadr** FRCSEng, FRCSEd(Orth)
Chairman, Orthopaedic Department, VA Medical Center, Washington. Assistant Professor, Georgetown University Hospital, Washington, U.S.A.

**Fabrizio Salimei** MD
Resident in Orthopaedic Surgery, Second University of Rome, Italy.

**John T. Scales** OBE, FRCS, CIMechE
Professor in Biomedical Engineering, University of London. Director, Department of Biomedical Engineering, Institute of Orthopaedics, Royal National Orthopaedic Hospital, Stanmore, Middlesex, U.K.

**S. V. Sharma** MSOrth
Reader, Department of Orthopaedics, Institute of Medical Sciences, Banaras Hindu University, Varamasi, India.

**Stephen N. Shaw** MSc
Research Associate, The Queen's University of Belfast, Musgrave Park Hospital, Belfast, U.K.

**Philip Shelley** PhD
Research Fellow and Biomechanical Engineer, Wrightington Hospital,

Lancashire, U.K.

**David Siu** PEng, MSc

Resident Engineer, Clinical Mechanics Group, Queen's University, Kingston, Ontario, Canada.

**R. B. Smith** BSc, FRCS

Consultant Orthopaedic Surgeon, Royal Preston Hospital, Preston, U.K.

**J. D. Spencer** MRCP, FRCS

Consultant Orthopaedic Surgeon, Guy's Hospital, London, U.K.

**A. Strover** FRCS

Consultant Orthopaedic Surgeon, Bromsgrove General Hospital, West Midlands.

Honorary Lecturer, Department of Orthopaedic Surgery, University of Birmingham, Oswestry, U.K.

**E. P. Szypryt** FRCS

Spinal Research Fellow and Orthopaedic Registrar, Department of Orthopaedics and Trauma Surgery, University Hospital, Queen's Medical Centre, Nottingham, U.K.

**Umberto Tarantino** MD

Orthopaedic Surgeon, Second University of Rome, Italy.

**N. J. Toff** BScHons, DRCOG

Medical Officer, The Travellers' Medical Service Limited, U.K.

**André Trifaud** MD

Professor of Orthopaedic Surgery and Chief of Service, Clinique Orthopedique et Traumatologie, Hopital de la Conception, Marseille, France.

**Naoichi Tsuyama** MD, DrMedSci

President, National Rehabilitation Center for the Disabled, Tokorozawa City.

Professor Emeritus, The University of Tokyo, Japan.

**S. M. Tuli** MS, PhD, FAMS

Professor of Orthopaedics and Director, Institute of Medical Sciences, Banaras Hindu University, Varamasi, India.

**Ettore Verni** MD

Resident, Department of Orthopaedic Surgery, Istituto Ortopedico Rizzoli, Bologna, Italy.

**D. I. Walker** FRCS

Consultant Orthopaedic Surgeon, Rochdale Infirmary, Rochdale, U.K.

**F. B. Webb** FRACS

Senior Visiting Orthopaedic Surgeon, Fremantle Hospital, Western Australia.

**B. G. Weber** MD

Chief of Service, Department of Orthopedics, Kantonsspital, St. Gallen, Switzerland.

**J. N. Wilson** ChM, FRCS

Honorary Consulting Orthopaedic Surgeon, Royal National Orthopaedic Hospital, Stanmore, Middlesex; National Hospital, London; and Department of Biomedical Engineering, Institute of Orthopaedics, London, U.K.

**Philip D. Wilson Jr** MD

Surgeon-in-Chief and Professor of Surgery (Orthopaedics), The Hospital for Special Surgery, The New York Hospital and Cornell University Medical College, New York, U.S.A.

**Winfried W. Winkelmann** MD

Professor of Orthopaedic Surgery, University of Dusseldorf, West Germany.

**Timothy M. Wright** PhD

Associate Scientist and Associate Professor of Applied Biomechanics (Surgery), The Hospital for Special Surgery and Cornell University Medical College, New York, U.S.A.

**B. Michael Wroblewski** FRCS

Consultant Orthopaedic Surgeon, Wrightington Hospital, Lancashire, U.K.

# 1. THE EVOLUTION OF ORTHOPAEDIC SURGERY BEFORE 1886

## J. R. Kirkup

As is well known, the French word 'orthopédie' translated as orthopaedia, was coined by Nicolas Andry in 1741, to encompass all children's deformities including cleft palate, abnormalities of the nails, hair and teeth, speech defects and many other disfigurements, no longer considered to be orthopaedic (Andry 1741). Andry, who also gave us the 'orthopaedic tree', was a professor of theology turned physician and a bitter opponent of surgeons. As Dean of the Medical Faculty in Paris, he obstructed the teaching of surgery by surgeons and, in particular hounded Jean Louis Petit, a surgeon of exceptional talent, inventor of the screw tourniquet, Fellow of the Royal Society of London and author of important works including a treatise on bone diseases (Petit 1705). In this latter work, Petit drew together the two limbs of trauma and disease, thus emphasising their interdependence, to the fury of Andry. Following a successful third edition in 1736, Petit was left in peace by Andry who then wrote his L'Orthopédie, perhaps in exasperation, for he was then 83 years old.

Other authors who combined locomotor trauma and disease in a single work included Alexis Boyer in 1803 and James Wilson in 1820; however these attempts to unify the study of orthopaedic surgery, as we now understand it, were not repeated until the 20th century, although in practice many surgeons worked in both fields. Thus, Hugh Owen Thomas, celebrated for systematic conservative management of orthopaedic disease and deformity, also treated fractures and was a competent, active general surgeon.

Broadly speaking, orthopaedic diagnosis is self-evident and readily agreed, whilst orthopaedic treatment provokes wide differences of opinion over alternative methods of management. Therefore, in the following brief analysis, it is proposed to examine the main branches of the orthopaedic "treatment-tree", still growing rapidly in response to various stimuli and best observed after its leaves have fallen.

To state that trauma, deformity and disease have accompanied man since his origin, is no speculation; certainly by the time of Hippocrates in 450 BC, fractures and dislocations already composed an extensive and precise branch of study, whereas bone and joint disease remained poorly defined until clarified by bacteriology and, by x-rays discovered when Sir Harry Platt was nine years old. This is not to indicate that 'cold' orthopaedic conditions were not treated, although their effective management was by splintage, counter-irritation and amputation until the 19th century, when certain discoveries revolutionised surgical practice. In particular, the introduction of anaesthesia by Morton in 1846 and of antiseptic wound management by Lister in 1867 rapidly expanded the surgeon's repertoire. However, true aseptic surgery had to await the thermal sterilisation of equipment introduced in Germany and France about 1882, although this was slow to be accepted in Britain. Nevertheless, by the time Sir Harry was a student, asepsis and Lane's 'no touch' technique were generally acknowledged.

For many centuries, fractures were secured with bandages impregnated with egg-white, flour, wine and so on, and applied after the complicated system of Hippocrates. This method persisted until the mid 19th century when plaster of Paris on bandages was introduced by Mathijsen in 1852 and other methods of control evolved. Although Lister demonstrated the successful silver wiring of fractures of the patella and olecranon, open reduction was rare before 1886. Surprisingly, continous traction for fractures was technically unsatisfactory until Buck introduced adhesive skin traction about 1860; earlier methods of bandage traction often resulted in the skin sloughing around the ankle, whilst skeletal traction is a 20th century concept. External fixation was initiated by Malgaigne in 1848 when he controlled patellar fractures with a pair of hooks held together by a compression screw. A further form of external fixation involved subcutaneous insertion of long steel nails or ivory pegs for non-union of tibial fractures.

It is a curious fact that before anaesthesia, books devoted to fractures and dislocations offered much more discussion on dislocations than fractures, indicating that the reduction of dislocated hips and shoulders, especially in muscular men, was often formidable in the absence of guaranteed muscle relaxation.   Following the introduction of anaesthesia, however, less and less space was given to dislocations, for as Erichsen noted in 1853, "In no department of practical surgery has the administration of anaesthetic agents been attended by more advantageous results".

In the 19th century, many fractures and indeed deformities, continued to be treated by amputation, despite the complications of stump infection and secondary haemorrhage leading to high mortality. Amputation, feared by the Greeks and reluctantly admitted by the Romans, was given impetus by the introduction of gun powder, although its general adoption was slow.   Even in the 17th century Woodall wrote in cautionary vein "....it is no small presumption to Dismember the Image of God" (Woodall 1617), and he advised strongly against amputation at the full moon.   Nevertheless, on ships and on the battlefield this procedure often seemed appropriate when limbs were badly shattered. However, it was the appalling results of amputation in hospitals which finally stimulated Lister to investigate antiseptic methods (Lister 1867).

Conservative management of deformity and disease embraced, and still does, a wide range of therapies including magic, faith as seen in cases of scrophula or Kings-evil (that is bovine tuberculosis, touched by Charles II), rest, movement, venesection, manipulation, massage, bathing (including the waters of the biblical Jordan) and acupuncture.   If the application of a cupping glass to the buttock for sciatica looks bizarre, it is little different and probably just as effective as other forms of counter-irritation, including radiant heat, ultra-sound and so on.   And splintage, discussed in detail by Francis Glisson in 1650 when he wrote the first treatise on rickets, the English disease, finally achieved unparalleled curative efficiency in the hands of H. O. Thomas in 1876.

In considering operative treatment, we enter the modern era of orthopaedic surgery.   Although sternomastoid tenotomy was performed by Minnius in 1685, it was club-foot tenotomy pioneered by Delpech in 1816 and developed scientifically by Stromeyer (1838) which stimulated a new approach to deformity and encouraged specialisation, resulting in the foundation of orthopaedic institutes and hospitals.   At the same time, sternomastoid tenotomy was revived and other techniques emerged.

Diseased joint excision or exsection reported by Park in 1781, was repeated occasionally before anaesthesia was available.   This technique often saved an amputation, whilst the best results achieved, fortuitously, a stable fusion; later, deliberate arthrodesis became an objective whilst in 1881 Albert introduced fusion to stabilise paralysed limbs.   The excision of one joint surface to create an arthroplasty developed at the same time and in 1860, Verneuil attempted the first interposition arthroplasty with muscle.

Barton's successful correction of knee-flexion contracture by wedge osteotomy in 1837 was followed by correction of knock knee in 1839 by Meyer who introduced the term osteotomy.   Utilising antiseptic technique, Macewen, who designed the osteotome, reported 1,800 corrective femoral osteotomies for rachitic knock-knees in 1884 without serious infection.

## CONCLUSION

The author is only too well aware of the deficiencies of this short account and regrets omitting various discoveries, several procedures and many famous men.   Despite this, it is evident that one hundred years ago, most fundamental orthopaedic operations had emerged and many were well established.

If, in Sir Harry's life-time aseptic technique, x-rays, blood transfusion, antibiotics, vaccines, stainless steel, internal fixation and replacement arthroplasty have altered the spectrum of orthopaedic surgery, they have not changed its direction;  and it is contended, that the active practitioners of 1886, such as Robert Jones, Louis Ombrédanne, Adolf Lorenz, Albin Lambotte, Fritz Lange, Ricardo Galeazzi, Robert Lovett, Murk Jansen and Arbuthnot Lane would not feel lost today, if they could only reappear before us.

## REFERENCES

Andry, N. (1741).  L'orthopédie ou l'art de prévenir et de corriger dans les enfants, les difformités du corps.  Alix, Paris.

Boyer, C. (1803).  Lecons.....sur les maladies des os.  (Ed. Richerand,

A.), Boyer, Paris.

Erichsen, J. (1853). The science and art of surgery.    Walton,    London,
p. 218.

Lister,    J.    (1867).    On    a    new    method of treating compound fracture,
abscess etc.    Lancet, 1:    326.

Petit, J. L. (1705). L'art de guérir    les    maladies    des    os.    Houry,
Paris.

Stromeyer,    G.    F.    L.    (1838).    Beitrage    zür    operativen    Orthopadik.
Helwing, Hanover.

Wilson, J. (1820).    Lectures on....the skeleton and on the    diseases    of
the bones and joints.    Burgess, London.

Woodall, J. (1617).    The surgions mate.    Lisle, London, pp. 172-5.

## 2. SIR HARRY PLATT AND SIR ROBERT JONES

### R. Owen

Young Harry first came under the spell of Robert Jones when he was taken unwillingly to Nelson Street to see the great man, Harry having injured the lower end of his femur in 1892 whilst living in Rochdale, and his knee having subsequently become very swollen. Sir Harry recalls how he immediately fell victim to the charm of the Master even though he hurt him terribly by injecting oil of turpentine into the joint. This was the beginning of a life-long relationship. There is little doubt that the course of orthopaedics in the United Kingdom was to some degree influenced by this early encounter. In his early teens, young Harry had to decide whether to pursue a medical career or enter the world of classical music. The decision was almost certainly made for him during his further visits to Nelson Street.

Sir Robert Jones' phenomenal career during the first quarter of this century and of his recognition as a Master Surgeon and Teacher in this country and abroad is well documented. During the second decade of this century Mr. Platt's career in Orthopaedic Surgery was also taking shape. Following graduation he flirted with a surgical career in London and worked as a House Surgeon at the Royal National Orthopaedic Hospital. In 1913, on the occasion of a meeting of the International Congress of Medicine in London, Robert Jones, already an international figure, invited the young Platt to the official dinner. Dr. Robert Lovatt gave the main speech of the evening. Those were heady days for the young man. From then onwards Harry Platt was inexorably drawn into the magic circle. During the First World War Major General Sir Robert Jones gathered around him a group of young men, Captain Platt amongst them, who were later despatched all over Great Britain to establish Orthopaedic Hospitals to care for the injured soldier and later crippled children. We should reflect briefly on some of his close colleagues in that team.    Tom MacMurray, whose widow previously Miss Evershed, Secretary to Sir Robert Jones, is still alive today at the age of 95, Gaythorn Girdlestone, Naughton Dunn, Alan Malkin, MacCrae Aitkin, Rowley Bristow, Elmsley, Fairbank, and Hey Groves, Maude Forrester Brown and last but not least Sir Robert's dearest pupil Noel Chavasse, V.C. and Bar, who fell in France:- and many others.    Sir Harry knew them all.

Harry Platt witnessed the birth of the British Orthopaedic Association at the Cafe Royal in 1918 and at Sir Robert's request was made First Secretary.    Sir Robert also encouraged him to travel in Europe and particularly in the United States, a young ambassador for British Orthopaedics.    His visits to North America may have sown the seed of the A.B.C. Exchange Travelling Fellowship.

In 1926 Sir Robert enlisted Harry to collaborate in the production of the second edition of that classic book by Jones and Lovatt, Sir Robert's great friend Lovatt having died in Liverpool the year previously.    Between 1926 and 1928 Sir Harry spent almost every weekend at Belvedere Road, Liverpool, working on "the book", his reward being that of good food and wine and increasing friendship.    Alas there was no third edition.

In 1921 Sir Robert established the Mastership Degree of Orthopaedic Surgery in the University of Liverpool.    As a mark of respect Sir Harry was made Honorary Member of the M.Ch.Orth. Society some years ago.

In 1929 S.I.C.O.T. came into being; although Sir Robert was luke-warm over the venture, Dr. Albee was keen.    The meeting was held in Paris in 1930; Sir Robert then aged 73 years was unanimously made President and Dr. Delchef Secretary.    At that meeting Mr. Platt should have been the British delegate but suffered from duodenal ulceration and so Thomas Fairbank deputised.

It was once said of Sir Robert Jones by his great friend Lord Moynihan "This extraordinary capacity for imbibing new ideas, always feeling there was something to learn put him in a class apart from other men of his generation".    A fair degree of the great man's philosophy has surely rubbed off on this pupil to whom this Festschrift is dedicated.

## 3. SIR HARRY PLATT AND ACCIDENT SERVICES IN BRITAIN

P. S. London

The dominant influence of orthopaedic surgeons in organizing the care of injured persons was established by Mr. Robert Jones when he set up a system that allowed the men injured while building the Manchester Ship Canal to be conveyed promptly to hospitals set up along its length. Some 20 years later Sir Robert Jones, resplendent in military uniform that did not entirely suit his avuncular appearance, took in hand not only the surgical treatment but also the rehabilitation of men wounded in the Kaiser's war.

The other dominant figure in organization of the care of injured persons was Sir Harry Platt. In 1914 he set up a fracture service at Ancoats Hospital, Manchester and he has gratefully acknowledged the support of his then surgical colleagues, Messrs. W. R. Douglas and J. Morley. This pioneering effort did not relieve Mr. Platt of the responsibility for general surgical undertakings, except, I understand, for abdominal emergencies.

The setting up of the full fracture service at Ancoats Hospital had to wait until after the war. In his description of the service in the Lancet in 1921, Mr. Platt stated that "segregation of fractures in a special service or subservice is an absolute necessity". He also separated their records from those dealing with diseases and in his address to the meeting of the British Medical Association in Bath in 1925 he stated that fractures should be "under the control of surgeons of full rank". He kept that control by means of his weekly fracture clinics, at which two secretaries took the dictated notes. In all this it is easy to recognize the most likely source of Gissane's policy and practices at the Birmingham Accident Hospital twenty years later (Gissane 1967). He separated the injured from the ill and provided continuity of care under the supervision of a consultant. It is a pleasure to record Sir Harry's support for what Gissane called the Birmingham experiment.

It is interesting to look back on those early days. One third of the 75 surgical beds at Ancoats Hospital were available to orthopaedic surgeons but most of the 30 or so new fractures that were seen each week were treated at home. The metal splints favoured by Liverpool were used in many cases; Thomas's splints and fixed traction were used for many fractures of the lower limb and – shades of Agnes Hunt's practice – these patients were conveyed to and from the fracture clinics, splints and all: Plaster of Paris was "occasionally employed for special purposes", mainly to maintain abduction at the shoulder and supination of the forearm.

Junior medical staff, with student masseuses and nurses in 'splint teams', did the donkey work in the fracture clinics. Physiotherapy began in the early weeks and it is interesting that the orthopaedic registrar was in charge of the physiotherapy department. Today, such an arrangement might be too much for Sir Harry, even at his most persuasive and insistent.

At the British Medical Association meeting Mr. Platt referred to the fact that Mr. Gask (of St. Bartholomew's Hospital) viewed "this scheme with misgivings" and, while he "did not question the sincerity of Mr. Gask's views", "his quixotic defence of a losing cause compelled admiration" (Platt 1925). One may wonder how much Mr. Gask appreciated that admiration and whether or not he shared the self-confident Mr. Platt's view that his cause was lost.

What Sir Harry has described as the battle for the take-over of fractures by orthopaedic surgeons succeeded to the extent that when he moved to the Manchester Royal Infirmary in 1934 it was agreed that he should take over all fractures and allied injuries.

Sir Harry has merely touched on his part in the setting up of the wartime Emergency Medical Service. This gave the teaching hospitals responsibility for supervising the medical services in related sectors of the country. It enabled them to evacuate patients from cities and to continue to exercise some control over their management in the receiving hospitals. It also gave students and staff an opportunity to get away from the bombing. It was easy for us youngsters to take it all for granted and not to recognize that it included perhaps the best accident service that Britain has ever had.

For those that are not steeped in orthopaedic tradition, Sir Harry Platt is perhaps best known for his chairmanship of the Subcommittee on Accident and Emergency Services of the Standing Medical Advisory Committee of the Central Health Services' Council, which quickly (and for obvious reasons) became known as the Platt committee. Unlike a number of other committees that had been reporting and recommending on the subject of Accident Services, the main recommendations of the Platt committee were implemented. The principles of 50 years before were still sound enough to be applied to the wider field of accident services.

Perhaps the earliest discernible effect was the replacement of signs bearing the words Casualty Department by signs bearing the words Accident and Emergency Department. The reason for this change was the committee's wish to emphasize that erstwhile casualty departments should concentrate on patients that needed prompt attention in hospital and should shed the burden of up to 50% of patients who could be dealt with by their general practitioners.

The Platt committee's recommendation that, as a general rule, orthopaedic surgeons would be the most appropriate specialists to take charge of accident and emergency departments was hailed by orthopaedic surgeons with approval, even enthusiasm, because there was still concern about the standards of care of many injuries. Within 10 years, however, that enthusiasm had largely evaporated, for the simple, but understandable, reason that the public had remained unaware of the reasons for the change of name. It is perhaps fair to add that even if the public had understood the reasons for the change they would have put their own convenience before the good intentions of Sir Harry and his subcommittee. The subcommittee's objective was admirable but Sir Harry has perhaps reflected with a rueful smile on the fact that the public's well developed sense of its own rights has brought more and more to hospitals with conditions that do not need any sort of medical attention. The complete frustration, in this respect, of the subcommittee's intentions is the reason why I continue to speak of casualty departments.

An important consequence of disillusionment of orthopaedic surgeons was the remark of the late Mr. Norman Capener at a meeting at the Ministry of Health in 1970 that, "What we want is a super GP", in casualty. Thus was born the process of accepting the recommendations of such men as Maurice Ellis and R. S. Garden that there should be casualty consultants.

For all the success of this new specialty in achieving consultant status, a training programme and higher diplomas it cannot be said that all is well with regard to the care of the injured and particularly the severely injured. The Royal College of Surgeons of England has instituted an enquiry into the advisability of establishing first class accident centres in which the severely injured will receive prompt attention under suitably skilled and experienced leadership. Professor Irving (1987) stated clearly the importance of establishing the facts upon which to base recommendations for improving the service and I am delighted by his remark that something like Gissane's service may be required. Years ago, Gissane advocated a national network of a dozen or more accident hospitals. Even if one substitutes 'service' for 'hospital' one comes up against the practical difficulties of ensuring the availability and the interest of suitably experienced men and women, not to mention the goodwill, that are essential if the necessary range of surgical and other participants is to be welded into a successful accident service. One may take severe head injuries as an example. They are often accompanied by serious injuries of other parts and require first intense and then prolonged care. Byrnes (1987) emphasized the need for general and orthopaedic surgeons to be trained in cranial surgery but it needs to be remembered that all head injuries require careful observation, some require timely reference for special care, but only a few require operations on the skull or brain. In the case of the physically or mentally crippled survivors the need is less for the attention of doctors than for that of the services allied to medicine and the support of the family. Awareness of these needs is in some ways more important than training in surgical techniques.

Things have changed since the building of the Manchester Ship Canal and the fracture service at Ancoats Hospital. Not only have injuries of the limbs become much more severe but severe injuries of the head and trunk are treatable with a degree of success that was inconceivable in those days. For these injuries anaesthetists and surgeons from more than one specialty are necessary. The methods have changed out of all recognition in the last 100 years but the principles have not.

It is ironic that when wiser minds are trying to decide how best to apply the policies of Sir Robert Jones, Sir Harry Platt and Professor Gissane to the care of severely injured persons, the South Birmingham Health District seems to be bent on terminating Gissane's Birmingham experiment.

## REFERENCES

Byrnes, D. P. (1987). Head Injuries. In: Current Trends in Orthopaedic Surgery. Festschrift to Sir Harry Platt, (Eds. Galasko, C. S. B. and Noble, J.). Manchester University Press, Manchester.

Gissane, W. (1967). The care of the injured. The development and purpose of an accident hospital. Annals of the Royal College of Surgeons of England, 41: 335-343.

Irving, M. H. (1987). The development of accident services. In: Current Trends in Orthopaedic Surgery. Festschrift to Sir Harry Platt, (Eds. Galasko C. S. B. and Noble J.). Manchester University Press, Manchester.

Platt, H. (1921). Organization of a fracture service. Lancet, ii: 620-621.

Platt, H. (1925). Address to British Medical Association meeting. British Medical Journal, ii: 325-326.

Report of the Subcommittee on Accident and Emergency Services (1962). Central Health Services Council Standing Medical Advisory Committee (Under the chairmanship of Sir Harry Platt). H.M.S.O., London.

# 4.THE TRANSATLANTIC CONNECTION

## Allan M. McKelvie

"One ship drives East and another West
With the self same winds that blow
T'is the set of the sails
And not the gales
Which tells us the way to go".

(From "The Winds of Fate" by Ella Wheeler Wilcox)

Harry Platt was a sail setter and a trend setter. He was the first Travelling Orthopaedic Fellow. For 73 years he was the Transatlantic Orthopaedic Ambassador extraordinaire. Of all the many things that he accomplished in Orthopaedics, one of the most auspicious was a Transatlantic Connection with enormous ramifications in peace and war. It started with his bold decision to visit the Massachusetts General Hospital in 1913, and meet the Boston pioneers of Orthopaedic Surgery. The Connection was established.

In 1917, prior to the U.S. entry into World War I, volunteer Orthopaedic Surgeons led by Robert Osgood from Boston, sailed to the United Kingdom. They were welcomed in Liverpool by Sir Robert and Lady Jones and went to work with the R.A.M.C. Some went north to the Edinburgh War Hospital, and some south to the Welsh Metropolitan Hospital, Cardiff. The Connection was strengthened in War.

The British Orthopaedic Association was born in London in 1917. Perhaps the "Midwife" was Robert Osgood of Boston. The Transatlantic Connection was "there at the creation." Over the years Robert Osgood was the Eastern terminal of the Translantic Connection.

Between the Wars Sir Harry was the very cynosure of International Orthopaedic activity. He held centre stage as Orthopaedics identified itself as a separate surgical entity, and was a founding member and later President of the International Federation of Surgical Colleges and S.I.C.O.T.

Later came the "Printed Connection" (The Journal of Bone and Joint Surgery) again through Boston.

A great and close friend of Sir Robert Jones was Lord Moynihan, who like Jones and Platt was a solid Americophile. He was the first President of the Royal College of Surgeons of England appointed from

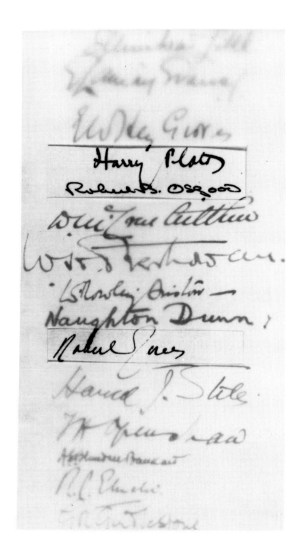

FIG. 1.   The signatures at the 1917 Cafe Royal Dinner when the British
Orthopaedic Assocation was born.

outside London.   Sir Harry was the second  and  the  first  Orthopaedic
Surgeon appointed President.

    In  World  War  I,  Dr.  Philip Wilson of Boston, and later New York,
volunteered to join  the  Harvard  unit  at  the  American  Hospital  in
Neuilly,  Paris.   A  youthful blond Boy Scout stretcher bearer in that
hospital was none other than Robert Merle D'Aubigne.   In World  War  II
as  a  member  of  the  Paris underground resistance he _just_ escaped the

Gestapo by 10 minutes, on his trusty bicycle.  In 1940 prior to the
U.S. entry into the War, Philip Wilson in New York organized, raised
funds for and led a volunteer unit of Orthopaedic Surgeons to work in
the American Hospital in Britain, first at Park Prewett and later at the
Churchill Hospital, Oxford.  He was awarded an O.B.E. for his
contribution to the War effort, and in correspondence he referred to
Harry Platt as "The Fairy Godfather" of the American Hospital in
Britain.  Once again the Transatlantic Orthopaedic Connection proved to
be a strong and noble bond, which was strengthened during the Second
World War.

Since the War that bond has grown ever stronger with Orthopaedic
Surgeons crossing the Atlantic regularly, bringing new techniques with
them and taking back new ideas.  The ABC Travelling Fellowship has
contributed significantly to that orthopaedic "Transatlantic Connection"
which had its beginning when Sir Harry visited Boston in 1913.

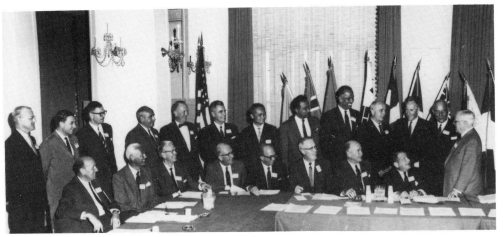

**INTERNATIONAL FEDERATION OF SURGICAL COLLEGES**
**1962 ANNUAL MEETING IN ATLANTIC CITY**

| K. CASSELS | E. HASNER | A. L. GOODALL | H. MILWIDSKY | CARL SEMB | K. R. INBERG | A. RAMIREZ | P. K. SEN |
|---|---|---|---|---|---|---|---|
| (U. K. ) | (Denmark) | (Glasgow) | (Israel) | (Norway) | (Finland) | (Philippines) | (India) |
| Secretary | | | | | | | |

| A. K. BASU | R. M. ZOLLINGER | FRANK GLENN | J. F. NUBOER | SIR HARRY PLATT |
|---|---|---|---|---|
| (India) | (U. S. A. ) | (U. S. A. ) | (Holland) | (U. K. ) |
| | | | | President |

| P. KYRLE | A. M. FEHR | FRITZ LINDER | W. C. BARBER | A. J. HELFET | W. C. MACKENZIE | SIR ARTHUR PORRITT | I. S. RAVDIN |
|---|---|---|---|---|---|---|---|
| (Austria) | (Switzerland) | (Germany) | (East Africa) | (South Africa) | (Canada) | (U. K. ) | (U. S. A. ) |
| | | | | | | | Vice-President |

FIG. 2.  The delegates of the International Federation of Surgical
Colleges in Atlantic City in 1962 recognize their President.  This
photograph reminds me of Oliver Goldsmith's Schoolmaster in "The
Deserted Village" 1770.
          "And still they gazed and still the wonder grew
          That one small head could carry all he knew"

# 5.OVERVIEW OF SHOULDER INSTABILITY – FROM PLATT TO THE PRESENT

Carter R. Rowe

Although Harry Platt has had many interests in his remarkable career in orthopaedic surgery, one of his earliest was instability of the shoulder.

Broca and Hartman in 1890, identified avulsion of the capsule and labrum from the rim of the glenoid as a cause of recurrent dislocation and in 1906 Perthes advocated repairing the capsule back to the rim. Bankart (1923) popularized Perthes' technique and pronounced the avulsed capsule as the one and only "essential" lesion of recurrent dislocation. There was no question that this was the basic problem of recurrent traumatic dislocations. However, as more unstable shoulders were explored, more questions arose. Bankart lesions were not always present. This disturbed the young orthopaedic surgeon from Manchester, and in the mid-twenties, he questioned Mr. Bankart of London as to what the surgeon should do, when, on exploring the shoulder for recurrent anterior dislocation, no "essential" lesion was present. Osmond-Clarke (1948) quoted Harry Platt's significant remarks, "I soon found out there was no single or constant Bankartian lesion capable of being repaired by a standard procedure. If there were instances of shoulder instability without the classic Bankart lesion, what technical procedure should be carried out?".

In 1925, Platt took a step beyond Broca and Hartman, Perthes and Bankart, and devised his own procedure for the shoulder, which, in his judgement, would bring stability to the shoulder, whether there was a Bankart lesion present or not. This new procedure was performed initially at Ancoats Hospital, Manchester, on November 13, 1925 (Osmond-Clarke 1948).

In looking back, there is no question that Platt's direct questioning, opened Pandora's box (Figure 1) with subsequent multiple

technical approaches for multiple "essential" lesions. It was evident
that repair of the shoulder for recurrent dislocation would never be the
same again! Procedure after procedure were reported for multiple new
causative lesions such as excess laxity of the capsule, Hill-Sachs
lesion of the humeral head, fracture of the glenoid rim, rupture of the
subscapularis muscle, variations in the size, shape and inclination of
the glenoid fossa, and few ill-defined "neuromuscular" abnormalities.

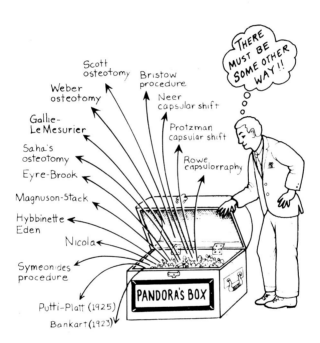

FIG. 1. Sir Harry Platt's question to Mr. Bankart opened Pandora's box
to multiple "essential" lesions, and multiple operative techniques.
Would corrective surgery ever be the same?

In the late 1950's, I reported a study of 500 primary, or initial,
shoulder dislocations seen in the emergency ward of the Massachusetts
General Hospital (Rowe 1956). From this investigation, we realized,
for the first time, that instability of the shoulder was a far more
complex problem than we had previously considered. In addition to the
various causative anatomical lesions, we were beginning to identify
variations and different categories of dislocations. The assignment to
specific categories began in the nineteen sixties. In 1969, I reported

on the _atraumatic_ category which differed in pathology, and in some instances in treatment, from the usual traumatic group (Rowe 1969). These were the shoulders that disturbed Harry Platt, and which Gallie referred to in 1948 as those produced by "no traumatism". Many of these, we found, responded to specific resistive exercises, rather than to surgery.

Also, in 1969, Blazina and Satzman reported their experience with recurrent _transient_ subluxations of the shoulder, or the "dead arm" syndrome, seen chiefly in athletes. Further studies of this syndrome (Rowe and Zarins 1981) revealed two categories: those patients who were aware of "a movement", or "slipping" of their shoulder when throwing or using their arm forcefully above shoulder level, and those who were _not_ aware of their shoulder slipping, only of a sudden "paralyzing" pain when attempting the same activities. Soon the shoulder recovered, but the abnormality became disturbingly recurrent. Of the fifty shoulders operated on in this group, thirty-two (64%) had traumatic Bankart lesions. The remainder had excessive laxity of the joint capsule.

In 1973, we reported an in-depth study of the _voluntary_ subluxators and dislocators. Perhaps Hippocrates had referred to this unusual performance in some individuals. His description is quite characteristic of voluntary dislocators, ".........or you may see people who are so humid (flabby) that when they choose, they can dislocate their joints without pain, and reduce them in like manner". Two important conclusions resulted from our 1973 report:

(1) Electromyographic study explained the mechanism of displacing the shoulder by suppressing one force-couple of the shoulder musculature, and activating another, to subluxate or dislocate the shoulder posteriorly, anteriorly, or inferiorly.

(2) Secondly, a small group of the voluntary dislocators had underlying emotional or personality problems. They were able to continue displacing their shoulder, usually for some personal gain or protection, in spite of well-performed surgical procedures. We cautioned that surgery on this small group of patients usually resulted in failure (Rowe et al. 1973).

In 1980, Neer and Foster reported a fifth category of shoulder instability, _the involuntary subluxators_ (Figure 2). In these patients, the supporting tissues became overstretched from repeated dislocations, allowing the shoulder to subluxate, or dislocate, in certain positions of the arm, or when merely carrying a package. The instability of many of these shoulders was multidirectional. The usual operative procedures for the traumatic, atraumatic, or transient instabilities were not so successful for this group. Specific types of capsulorrhaphy proved more effective (Neer and Foster 1980, Protzman 1980, Rowe and Zarins 1981). Twenty-five to 30% of patients in this category responded initially to specific resistive exercises, eliminating the need for surgery.

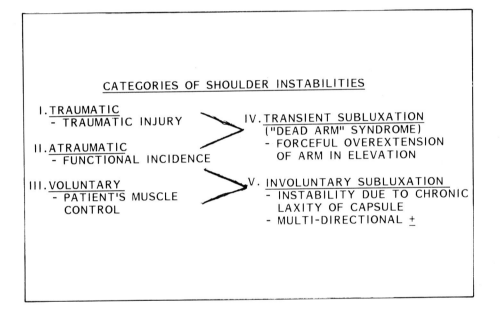

FIG. 2.    The five different categories of shoulder instability.

Thus, at the present time, the common, undistinguished recurrent dislocation of the shoulder of the past, is now a challenging and subtle instability complex of six causative lesions, and five different categories (Figure 3). Although many of the problems of shoulder instability have been analyzed, many, to date, remain unsolved.

All of which brings us full circle back to Sir Harry Platt's questioning of Mr. Bankart, that there were problems of instability of the shoulder, other than the one "essential" lesion, and we, as surgeons, should acknowledge this and do something about it.

## INSTABILITIES OF THE SHOULDER

### 5 CATEGORIES

1. TRAUMATIC
2. ATRAUMATIC
3. TRANSIENT
4. VOLUNTARY
5. INVOLUNTARY

### 6 CAUSATIVE LESIONS

#### CAPSULE

1. AVULSION FROM RIM (BANKART LESION)
2. EXCESSIVE LAXITY

#### BONE

3. HILL-SACHS LESION
4. FRACTURE GLENOID RIM
5. VARIATIONS IN GLENOID TILT

#### MUSCLE

6. RUPTURE

THERE IS NO ONE "ESSENTIAL" LESION

FIG. 3. At present shoulder instability is a complex of five categories and six causative anatomical lesions.

This overview may be summarized in Sir Harry's inimitable words from his "Days with Sir Robert" – "I hope you will perceive that I am looking back to tomorrow".

## REFERENCES

Bankart, A. S. B. (1923). Recurrent or habitual dislocation of the shoulder. British Medical Journal, 2, 1132.

Blazina, M. E. and Satzman, J. S. (1969). Recurrent anterior subluxation of the shoulder in athletes – a distinct entity. Journal of Bone and Joint Surgery, 51-A, 1037-1038.

Broca, A. and Hartman, H. (1890). Contribution a l'etude des luxations de l'espanle.  Bulletin of the Society of Anatomy. SME Series, 4, 416-423.

Gallie, W. E. and LeMesurier, A. B. (1948).  Recurring dislocation of the shoulder. Journal of Bone and Joint Surgery, 30-B:  9-18.

Hippocrates (Translated by Adams). The Genuine Works of Hippocrates. (1946).  William and Wilkins, Baltimore, pp. 205-215.

Neer, C. S. II and Foster, C. R. (1980).  Inferior capsular shift for involuntary inferior and multidirectional instability of the shoulder. A preliminary report. Journal of Bone and Joint Surgery, 62-A, 897-908.

Osmond-Clarke, H. (1948).  Habitual dislocation of the shoulder – the Putti-Platt operation. Journal of Bone and Joint Surgery, 30-B, 19-25.

Perthes, G. (1906).  Uber operationen der Habituellen Shullerluxation. Deutsche Zeitschrift Fur Chirurgie, 85, 199.

Protzman, R. R. (1980).  Anterior instability of the shoulder.  Journal of Bone and Joint Surgery, 62-A, 909-918.

Rowe, C. R. (1956).  Prognosis in dislocation of the shoulder.  Journal of Bone and Joint Surgery, 38-A:  957-977.

Rowe, C. R. (1969).  Complicated dislocations of the shoulder. Guidelines in treatment. American Journal of Surgery, 117, 549-553.

Rowe, C. R., Pierce, D. S. and Clarke, J. (1973).  Voluntary dislocation of the shoulder. A preliminary report on a clinical, electromyographic and psychiatric study of twenty-six patients. Journal of Bone and Joint Surgery, 55-A, 445-460.

Rowe, C. R. and Zarins, B. (1981).  Recurrent transient subluxation of the shoulder. Journal of Bone and Joint Surgery, 63-A:  863-872.

## 6. RECURRENT DISLOCATION OF THE SHOULDER JOINT

G. Blatter
B. G. Weber

### INTRODUCTION

There are several causes of recurrent dislocation of the shoulder:

(i)   A congenital dysplasia of the glenoid cavity.  The result is a voluntary, playful habitual shoulder dislocation of the child.

(ii)  Paralysis of the shoulder muscles.  Due to the lack of muscle pull, the head of the humerus is dislocated inferiorly because of the pull of gravity of the arm.

(iii) By far the most frequent cause is trauma.  This is especially the case for anterior dislocations.

(iv)  Posterior dislocation may be caused by tetanic contractures such as seizures or electric accidents.

More than 250 operations have been devised for the treatment of recurrent dislocations of the shoulder.  All these operations may be divided into six categories.

(i)   Operations on the joint capsule.

(ii)  Fastening procedures using fascia etc.

(iii) Muscle insertion transfers.

(iv)  Operations on the humeral head or the glenoid.

(v)   Operations on the glenoid rim.

(vi)  "Unconventional" procedures.

In order to treat shoulder dislocations appropriately the pathologic-anatomical alterations must be taken into account.  In the common, recurrent anterior dislocations caused by trauma the following pathological lesions may be present (Figure 1).

(i)   An enlarged joint capsule and a stretched subscapularis muscle.

(ii)  The Bankart-lesion, which is a lesion of the glenoid rim.

(iii) The Malgaigne-or Hill-Sachs-lesion, which is an

impression fracture of the humeral head and occurs at the first dislocation.

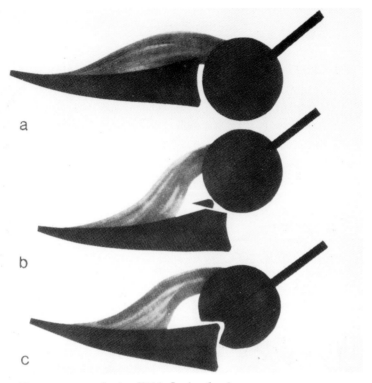

FIG. 1. The anatomy of the Hill-Sachs-lesion.
The right shoulder is seen in horizontal crossection.
(a)   An uninjured shoulder. The subscapularis muscle is not over-
      stretched despite the external rotation as drawn here.
(b)   Dislocation and damage of the anterior rim of the glenoid.   The
      subscapularis muscle is overstretched.
(c)   Dislocation and impaction of the posterior aspect of the humeral
      head.   The subscapularis muscle is overstretched.

Over 80% of all recurrent dislocating shoulders have a major Hill-Sachs-lesion, seen either on x-ray or intra-operatively. About 30 to 40% demonstrate a Bankart-lesion either in isolation or in addition to a Hill-Sachs-lesion.

These two different bony lesions determine our surgical technique and not the capsular instability which is caused by the dislocation rather than causing the dislocation itself.

The goal of the operation is to prevent further dislocations and to retain normal mobility of the joint, without limiting external rotation.

The authors carry out that operation which will correct the specific anatomic lesion.


## SURGICAL TECHNIQUES


### Labrum-reconstruction and shortening of the subscapularis muscle (Figure 2).

Through a deltopectoral approach the tendon of the subscapularis is transsected just proximal to its insertion to the lesser tubercle. The joint is then opened and inspected. The avulsed fragment of the labrum is reattached by two or three screws after the rim of the glenoid has been freshened with an osteotome. The rim of the glenoid is

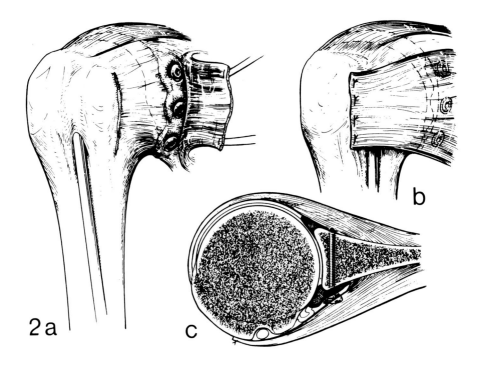

FIG. 2.    Labrum  reconstruction  and  tightening of the subscapularis muscle.
The right shoulder is viewed from in front and above.
(a)    The subscapularis muscle is detached and reflected.    The free labrum is screwed to the rim of the glenoid.
(b)    The subscapularis muscle is brought over the bicipital tendon and fixed to the greater tubercle.
(c)    The reattached labrum and the tightened subscapularis muscle.

reconstructed to prevent future dislocations.   The subscapularis muscle
is   shortened   by   1·5cm   either   by doubling or transferring the muscle
insertion to the greater tubercle.    The shortening of   the   muscle   and
tightening  of  the  capsule  is  to  correct   the laxity, caused by the
dislocation, and not to limit external rotation.

## The insertion of a bone graft (Figure 3).

If neither a Hill—Sachs—lesion nor a Bankart—lesion is the primary cause
for  the  dislocation,  glenoid  dysplasia or a posterior dislocation is
usually found.    After the  joint  has  been  opened  and  inspected,  a
corticocancellous bone graft is fixed to the neck of the scapula.    This
bone graft is placed extraarticularly either anteriorly  or   posteriorly
depending  on  the  direction of the dislocation and is fixed by screws.
The bone graft is taken from  the  iliac  wing.    The  subscapular  and
infraspinatus muscles  are  then  reapproximated  without shortening to
avoid any limitation of external rotation.

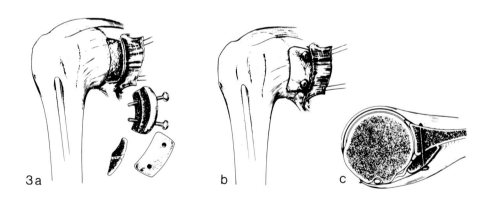

3a                          b                    c

FIG. 3.    Insertion of a bone graft.
The right shoulder is viewed from above and in front.
(a)    The subscapularis muscle is detached and turned back.    The neck
       of the scapula is freshened.    The corticocancellous bone graft
       which is taken from the iliac wing is freshened and fixed with
       two lagscrews.
(b)    The bone graft is screwed onto the neck of the scapula.
(c)    The bone graft lies extraarticularly and is more prominent than
       the osseous rim of the glenoid.    The subscapularis insertion is
       moved towards the greater tubercle to tighten the muscle.

Shortening of the subscapularis muscle with  osteotomy  of  the  humerus
(Figure 4).

Through  a  deltopectoral  incision  the proximal part of the humerus is
exposed from the lesser tubercle to the insertion of the deltoid muscle.
The   subscapularis   tendon   and   the  capsule  are  divided  and  the
glenohumeral  joint  is  inspected.   By  rotating   the   humerus   a
Hill-Sachs-lesion at the postero-lateral aspect of the humeral head  can

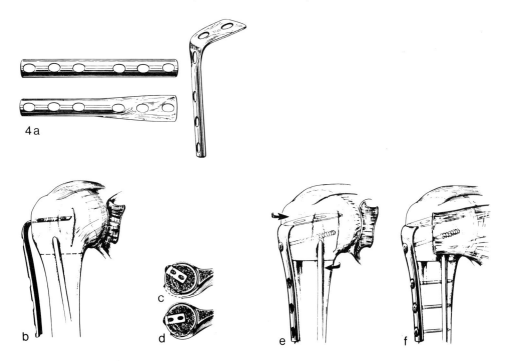

FIG. 4.    Advancement  of  the  subscapularis  muscle  and  rotational
osteotomy of the proximal humerus.  The right shoulder  is  viewed  from
above and in front.
(a)   One end of a 6 hole semitubular plate is flattened and bent into
      the shape of a blade plate.
(b)   Insertion of the blade plate into the humeral head from posterior
      to anterior, angled about 20 to 25° to the coronal plane.
(c)   Direction of the blade plate before osteotomy.
(d)   Direction of the blade plate after osteotomy.   The humeral head
      is internally rotated about 20 to 25°.
(e)   The osteotomy is completed, the plate is fixed to the humeral
      head with an additional screw, and the head is internally
      rotated.
(f)   The plate is fixed to the humeral shaft using the dynamic
      compression technique, and the insertion of the subscapularis
      muscle is moved laterally.

often be found.   The joint is opened and the glenoid rim and labrum are inspected for any lesions.   After the subcapital osteotomy the head  of the humerus is  internally rotated 20 to 25°.   The osteotomy is fixed with a six or seven hole semitubular plate, which is bent into the shape of a blade plate.   The tendon of the subscapularis muscle is shortened by doubling over or advancing it to the greater tubercle.

This operation is similar to  the  technique  described  by  Magnuson (1945) but  the  rotational  osteotomy avoids the decrease in mobility. One theoretical disadvantage is a  slight  loss  of  internal  rotation. However, this is less than 15°, which has no clinical effect.

## REFERENCES

Bankart, A. S. B. (1923).   Recurrent or habitual dislocation of the shoulder joint.  British Medical Journal, 2:  1132-1133.

Bankart, A. S. B. (1938). The  pathology  and  treatment  of  recurrent dislocation of  the  shoulder  joint.   British Journal of Surgery, 26: 23-29.

Dickson, J. W. and Devas, M. B. (1957).  Bankart's  operation  for recurrent dislocation of  the  shoulder.  Journal  of  Bone and Joint Surgery, 39-B:  114-119.

Eden, R.  (1920).   Zur  operativen  Behandlung  der  habituellen Schulterluxation. Zentralblatt fur Chirurgie, 47:  1002-1005.

Hill,  H. A. and Sachs, M. D. (1940).  The grooved defect of the humeral head.  A frequently unrecognized complication  of  dislocations  of  the shoulder joint.  Radiology, 35:  690-700.

Hovelius,  L.,  Thorling,  J. and Fredin, H. (1979).  Recurrent anterior dislocation of the shoulder.  Results after the Bankart and  Putti-Platt operations.  Journal of Bone and Joint Surgery, 61-A:  566-569.

Hovelius,  L.,  Korner,  L.,  Lundberg,  B., Åkermark, C., Herberts, P., Wredmark, T. and Berg, E. (1983).  The coracoid transfer  for  recurrent

dislocation  of the shoulder.   Technical aspects of the Bristow—Laterjet
procedure.   Journal of Bone and Joint Surgery, 65-A:   926-934.

Hybbinette, S. (1932).   De la transplantation d'un fragment osseux   pour
remédier  aux  luxations  récidivantes  de  l'épaule;   constatations et
resultants opératoires.   Acta Chirurgica Scandinavica, 71:   411-445.

Magnuson, P. B. (1945).   Treatment  of  recurrent  dislocation  of  the
shoulder.   Surgical Clinics of North America, 25:   14-20.

Magnuson,  P.  B. and Stack, J. K. (1943).   Recurrent dislocation of the
shoulder.   Journal of the American Medical Association, 123:   889-892.

Osmond—Clarke, H. (1948).   Habitual dislocation of  the  shoulder.   The
Putti-Platt operation.   Journal of Bone and Joint Surgery, 30-B:   19-25.

Weber,   B.   G.   (1979).   Die  gewohnheitsmässige  Schulterverrenkung.
Unfallkeilkunde, 82:   413-417.

# 7

RECURRENT ANTERIOR DISLOCATION OF THE SHOULDER TREATED BY SCAPULAR   NECK
OSTEOTOMY AND ANTERIOR BONE BLOCK THROUGH THE AXILLA.

S. M. Tuli
S. V. Sharma

## INTRODUCTION

Despite a voluminous literature on recurrent anterior dislocation of the
shoulder, the aetiology, pathogenesis and optimum methods of  management
are still not fully known.   Most of the operative techniques in current
use share a common  disadvantage  of  limitation  of  external  rotation
(Collins and Wilde 1973).

The  purpose  of this study was to evaluate a relatively new surgical
technique utilising  an axillary approach.


## PATIENTS AND METHODS

Thirteen (12 male and 1 female) young adults  suffering  from  recurrent
anterior  dislocation  of shoulder who attended the University Hospital,
Banaras Hindu University, Varanasi, during the period 1979 to 1985  were
evaluated.    Only  those  patients  who had at least three episodes of
recurrent dislocation were considered for the  study.    Young  patients
with  no history of epilepsy, addiction to drugs or other psycho-somatic
ailments were preferred.   The post-surgical follow-up ranged  from  two
to six years.

### Operative Technique

The  shoulder  was  approached  through  an  axillary approach (Tuli and
Sharma 1986).   A linear incision about 5cm long was made  perpendicular
to  the  posterior  áxillary  fold,  medial to the level of the shoulder
joint and parallel to the skin crease.   By blunt dissection  the  loose
areolar tissue was undermined and the subscapularis muscle  was exposed.

This was retracted by passing a bone lever behind the muscle, reaching
the upper border of the scapula lateral to the base of the coracoid
process. The following structures were then identified – anterior
margin of the glenoid, infraglenoid tubercle, the origin of the long
head of triceps muscle, teres minor muscle, and the axillary border of
the scapula. The periosteum was then raised from the front of the neck
of the scapula. The proposed line of osteotomy, parallel to the
anterior glenoid margin was marked, and the neck of scapula was
osteotomised. The osteotomy site was prized open and an autologous
cortico-cancellous bone graft, 3cm x 1·5cm and triangular in cross
section, was taken from the iliac crest and placed such that about
1·0cm of the graft projected antero-inferiorly. The graft was secured
and held under compression, as the osteotomes were gradually removed.
No suction drainage or blood transfusion was required. The wound was
closed with skin sutures, and the limb immobilised, with the shoulder in
flexion, adduction and internal rotation for 3 weeks. Active exercises
of the shoulder were then encouraged.


## RESULTS

There were no recurrences of dislocation following surgery and all the
patients returned to their original profession. All the patients
regained a full functional range of movement within 6 months of
operation except for two.. One had gross restriction of shoulder
movements and the other had 15° active external rotation and 80°
abduction.


## DISCUSSION

Bristow's procedure as reported by Helfet (1958) retained full function
of the shoulder and consisted of an anterior bone block occasioned by
transferring the coracoid process with its attached muscle origins
through subscapularis to the bare neck of the scapula. Lombardo and
co-authors (1976) reported a 2% recurrence in 51 patients operated upon
by Bristow's technique. It was further stated that none of the
athletes could return to their original level of performance. Eden

(1920) and Hybbinette (1932) independently described an operation wherein an autologous bone graft was placed against the anterior aspect of the neck of the scapula and rim of the glenoid cavity in a subperiosteal pocket to form an anterior wall or buttress of bone.

The surgical technique evaluated in the current study has the following advantages:-

(i)    The approach is extracapsular and joint movements are largely retained.

(ii)   The axillary approach through the intermuscular planes gives easy access to the front of scapula.

(iii)  The musculo-tendinous apparatus around the shoulder is minimally disturbed.

(iv)   The combination of an anterior bone block and redirectional osteotomy of the neck of the scapula increases the functional depth of the glenoid cavity in addition to the anterior buttress action.

(v)    The procedure is useful in all the age groups and is compatible with all sporting activities.


## REFERENCES

Collins, H. R. and Wilde, A. H. (1973). Shoulder instability in athletes. Orthopaedic Clinics of North America, 4: 759-774.

Eden, R. (1920). Zur operativen behandlung der habituellen schulterluxation (Operative treatment of habitual dislocation of the shoulder). Zentralblatt fur Chirurgie, 47: 1002-1005.

Helfet, A. J. (1958). Coracoid transplantation for recurring dislocation of the shoulder. Journal of Bone and Joint Surgery, 40-B: 198-202.

Hybbinette, S. (1932). De la transplantation d'un fragment osseux pour remedier aux luxations recidivantes de l'epaule constatation et resultats operatoires. Acta Chirurgica Scandinavica, 71: 411.

Lombardo, S. J., Kerlan, R. K., Jobe, F. W., Carter, V. S., Blazina, M.

E. and Shields, C. L. (1976). The modified Bristow procedure for recurrent dislocation of the shoulder. Journal of Bone and Joint Surgery, 58-A: 256-261.

Tuli, S. M. and Sharma, S. V. (1986). Axillary approach to the front of the shoulder and neck of the scapula. Indian Journal of Orthopaedics, 20: 211-213.

# 8

# THE MODIFIED STAPLE CAPSULORRHAPHY FOR THE SURGICAL CORRECTION OF RECURRENT ANTERIOR DISLOCATION OF THE SHOULDER

J. P. Hodgkinson
D. B. Case

## INTRODUCTION

More than 150 operations to stabilise recurrent anterior dislocation of the shoulder have been described. Probably the two most popular techniques are the Bankart repair (1938) and the Putti-Platt repair as described by Osmond-Clarke in 1948, their failure rates ranging from 0-13% (Adams 1948, Eyre Brook 1948, Watson Jones 1948, Dickson and Devas 1957, Brav 1960, Rowe 1963, Morrey and Janes 1976).

In 1931 Fouché (Du Toit and Roux 1956) performed the first staple capsulorrhaphy to correct recurrent anterior dislocaton of the shoulder. In the original staple capsulorrhaphy, the staples were inserted intracapsularly and there was no deliberate shortening of the subscapularis muscle; the reported failure rate was about 4% (Du Toit and Roux 1956, Boyd and Hunt 1965).

The modified staple capsulorrhaphy corrects the "Bankart lesion" and shortens subscapularis by the use of an extracapsular staple. This paper describes the operative technique of the modified staple capsulorrhaphy, and reviews the results in 29 patients who underwent this operation between 1970 and 1985.

## PATIENTS AND METHODS

During the period November 1970 to September 1985, 31 patients (24 male and 7 female) were treated for recurrent anterior dislocation of the shoulder by the modified staple capsulorrhaphy procedure. Their ages ranged from 18 years to 68 years with an average age of 27·3 years.

Twenty-nine patients could be contacted and were reviewed; the other two patients were untraceable and presumably have moved away from the area.

The time from first dislocation to surgery ranged from 5 months to 9 years with an average of 2·7 years. For most patients, the first dislocation was associated with moderate to severe trauma; the type of injury is shown in Figure 1.

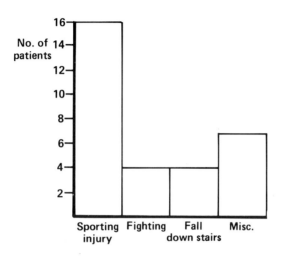

Type of injury at time of first dislocation

FIG. 1. Histogram showing the type of injury at the time of the first anterior dislocation, and the number of patients in each group.

Subsequent dislocations were caused by much less severe trauma. In four patients one of their dislocations was associated with axillary nerve dysfunction, but they had all fully recovered before surgery was undertaken. One patient suffered a greater tuberosity fracture at the time of his first dislocation.

Operative Technique

Under general anaesthetic, the patient was placed supine with a sand bag between the scapulae. The arm was towelled to allow its free movement. The incision was made from just below the lateral aspect of the clavicle, over the coracoid process and in the line of the delto-pectoral groove as far as the axillary fold. The delto-pectoral groove was developed and the cephalic vein was usually ligated. The coracoid process was then exposed and the conjoined tendon of coraco-brachialis and the short head of biceps identified. The interval between the conjoint tendon and pectoralis minor was opened taking care to avoid damage to the musculo-cutaneous nerve, the conjoint tendon freed and then divided about one centimetre from the tip of the coracoid process.

The arm was fully externally rotated, the upper and lower margins of subscapularis identified and subscapularis and the capsule were divided vertically at the level of the glenoid. The shoulder joint and anterior margin of the glenoid were inspected and the pathology identified. If a "Bankart lesion" was present the neck of the glenoid was 'rawed' prior to insertion of the staple. Using the staple holder (Figure 2), a staple was passed through the lateral cuff of subscapularis and the capsule, and with the arm then internally rotated, the staple was secured into the neck of the glenoid (Figure 3).

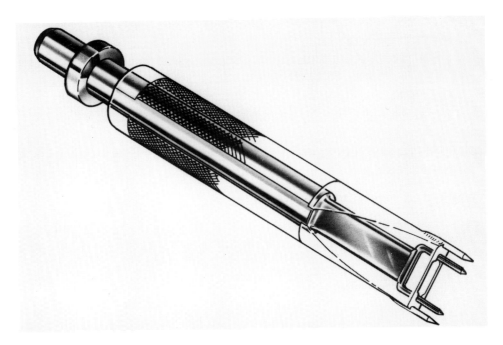

FIG. 2.   A diagramatic representation of the staple holder, punch and staple.

The medial cuff of subscapularis and the capsule were reefed as in the "Putti-Platt" repair, suturing them to the tendinous insertion of subscapularis.

The conjoint tendon of coraco-brachialis and the short head of biceps was resutured to the coracoid process, and the wound was closed in

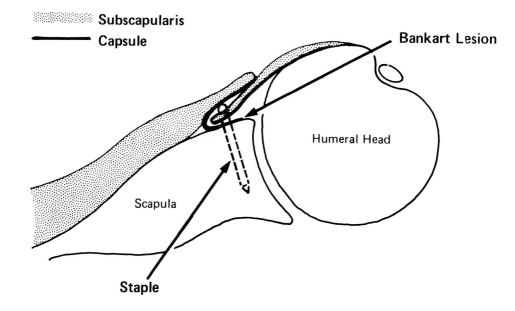

FIG. 3.    A cross-sectional diagram of a shoulder demonstrating the position of the staple and reefing of the medial cuff of the capsule and subscapularis.

layers after careful haemostasis.

Post operative management

The skin sutures were removed at 14 days.    The arm was rested in a sling for 6 weeks with an additional body bandage for the first 3 weeks. Mobilisation of the shoulder commenced at 6 weeks but the patients were advised to restrict their activities for a total of 3 months.


RESULTS


The follow-up ranged from 1 year to 15 years with an average of 5·5 years.    The 29 patients were assessed in terms of symptoms, activity, radiographic appearance, range of movement and complications.

Symptoms and Activity

The patients were asked to complete a questionnaire before being reviewed.   The results are shown in Table I.

TABLE I

Symptoms and Activity

|  | Yes | No |
|---|---|---|
| Have you returned to work? | 28 | 1 |
| How soon did you return? | 4 weeks to 6 months<br>Average time = 3·7 months | |
| Do you play sport? | 16 | 13 |
| Do you have any pain? | 9 | 20 |
| Are you pleased with the operation? | 28 | 1 |

The answers given by the twenty-nine patients in response to the questionnaire.

The one patient who was not working had rheumatoid arthritis and had retired before surgery was undertaken.   On average patients had returned to work 3·7 months after surgery.   Of the 16 patients involved in regular sport, 4 went swimming and 5 played racket sports, 3 of whom used the racket in the hand of their affected shoulder.

Nine patients reported occasional pain in their shoulder but only one was of any significance.   Three reported that they had slight discomfort if they slept on the affected side and 5 reported an occasional ache after heavy work.   There was one patient who complained of a continuous ache in her shoulder and she was the only patient not pleased with the operation.

Radiographic appearance

Radiographic examination showed that the staple remained satisfactory in 28 patients with no evidence of loosening or infection.   In one patient the staple had backed out completely, but this was noted 3 months after surgery and he had continued in demolition work, with no apparent problem.

Range of movement

External rotation was restricted in all patients when compared with their opposite shoulder.    The decrease in external rotation ranged from 10° to 50° with an average of 28°.    Five patients demonstrated a slight reduction in abduction (maximum 30°) and 8 patients had slightly restricted extension (maximum 20°).

## Complications

There have been no neurovascular problems and no further dislocations after surgery.

The only complication has been in the patient who complained of pain in the shoulder following surgery.    It may be that she had a low grade infection even though the wound has remained well healed and her blood parameters have been normal.    Removal of the staple is proposed.

## DISCUSSION

Anterior dislocation of the shoulder is a common injury and, probably more than any other joint, is subject to recurrence.    The age of the patient at the time of the primary dislocation has been shown to be the most important and consistent factor in determining recurrence (Rowe 1956).    In patients under 20 years of age, recurrence occurs in about 90% of cases (McLaughlin and Cavallaro 1950, Rowe and Sakellarides 1961, Henry and Genung 1982).    At any age recurrent anterior dislocation of the shoulder severely interferes with work and sporting activities.

The pathogenesis of recurrent anterior dislocation is probably multifactorial (Saha 1971, Morley and Janes 1976).    Although a "Hill-Sachs" or "Bankart" lesion is often present, there usually is considerable laxity within the anterior joint capsule (Rowe et al. 1984), and it is for this reason that it is justifiable to shorten the subscapularis muscle (Osmond Clarke 1948, Symeonides 1972).    The modified staple capsulorrhaphy procedure combines the repair of a detached anterior labrum with shortening of the subscapularis muscle. Technically it is a much easier procedure than many others described, and although some authors condemn the use of metal implants such as staples and screws in the vicinity of the shoulder joint, in this procedure the staple is placed extracapsularly and the joint is no more at risk than if a screw is used to secure an osteotomized coracoid process.

The staple holder was designed by one of the authors (D. B. C.) and can be adapted for use with the more modern barbed staples. This holder allows leverage of the lateral cuff of the capsule and subscapularis over the anterior rim of the glenoid; it ensures stability of the staple whilst positioning, and the punch aids easy and accurate insertion.


## CONCLUSION

The modified staple capsulorrhaphy is a technically easier procedure than many of the others described to correct recurrent anterior dislocation of the shoulder. It reduces operating time yet produces comparable long-term results and is without serious complication.


## ACKNOWLDGEMENTS

We would like to thank Mrs. Elizabeth Newton for typing this manuscript and the Medical Illustration Departments at the Royal Preston Hospital and Hope Hospital for the photographs and illustrations.


## REFERENCES

Adams, J. C. (1948). Recurrent dislocation of the shoulder. Journal of Bone and Joint Surgery, 30-B: 26-38.

Bankart, A. S. B. (1938). The pathology and treatment of recurrent dislocation of the shoulder joint. British Journal of Surgery, 26: 23-29.

Boyd, H. B. and Hunt, H. L. (1965). Recurrent dislocation of the shoulder: the staple capsulorrhaphy. Journal of Bone and Joint Surgery, 47-A: 1514-1520.

Brav, E. A. (1960). Recurrent dislocation of the shoulder: ten years experience with the Putti Platt reconstruction procedure. American Journal of Surgery, 100: 423-430.

Dickson, J. W. and Devas, M. B. (1957). Bankart's operation for recurrent dislocation of the shoulder. Journal of Bone and Joint Surgery, 39-B: 114-119.

Du Toit, G. T. and Roux, D. (1956). Recurrent dislocation of the shoulder: A twenty four year study of the Johannesburg stapling operation. Journal of Bone and Joint Surgery, 38-A: 1-12.

Eyre-Brook, A. L. (1948). Recurrent dislocation of the shoulder: lesions discovered in seventeen cases, surgery employed and intermediate report on results. Journal of Bone and Joint Surgery, 30-B: 39-46.

Henry, J. H. and Genung, J. A. (1982). Natural history of glenohumeral dislocation - revisited. American Journal of Sports Medicine, 10 135-137.

McLaughlin, H. L. and Cavallaro, W. U. (1950). Primary anterior dislocation of the shoulder. American Journal of Surgery, 80: 615-621.

Morrey, B. F.and Janes, J. M. (1976). Recurrent anterior dislocation of the shoulder. Long-term follow up of the Putti-Platt and Bankart procedures. Journal of Bone and Joint Surgery, 58-A: 252-256.

Osmond-Clark, H. (1948). Habitual dislocation of the shoulder: the Putti-Platt operation. Journal of Bone and Joint Surgery, 30-B: 19-25.

Rowe, C. R. (1956). Prognosis in dislocations of the shoulder. Journal of Bone and Joint Surgery, 38-A: 957-977.

Rowe, C. R. (1963). The results of operative treatment of recurrent dislocations of the shoulder. Surgical Clinics of North America, 43: 1667-1670.

Rowe, C. R. and Sakellarides, H. T. (1961). Factors related to recurrences of anterior dislocations of the shoulder. Clinical Orthopaedics and Related Research, 20: 40-48.

Rowe, C. R., Zarins, B. and Ciullo, J. V. (1984).  Recurrent anterior dislocation of the shoulder after surgical repair.  Apparent  causes  of failure  and  treatment.  Journal  of  Bone  and  Joint  Surgery,  66-A: 159-168.


Saha, A. K. (1971).  Dynamic stability of the gleno-humeral joint.  Acta Orthopaedica Scandinavica, 42:  491-505.


Symeonides,  P. P. (1972).  The significance of the subscapularis muscle in the pathogenesis of recurrent anterior dislocation of  the  shoulder. Journal of Bone and Joint Surgery, 54-B:  476-483.


Watson-Jones,  R. (1948).  Note on recurrent dislocation of the shoulder joint:  superior  approach  causing  the  only  failure  in  fifty  two operations  for  repair  of the labrum and capsule.  Journal of Bone and Joint Surgery, 30-B:  49-52.

# 9.THE UNSTABLE SHOULDER – A CT STUDY

M. Baratelli
M. Parrini

## INTRODUCTION

The causes of shoulder instability are multifactorial, no single anatomical lesion, soft tissue or bone, is responsible for every episode of recurrent anterior dislocation of the shoulder.  It is a result of a combination of traumatic factors and resulting forces expended at the weakest point of the shoulder.

Since an attempt is being made to rationalize the Bankart, modified Bristow, Magnusson–Stack, and Putti-Platt operations, different diagnostic procedures have been proposed as helpful adjuncts in substantiating the diagnosis and in planning the choice of treatment and surgical reconstruction (Symeonides 1972, DePalma 1973, Saha 1981, Turkel et al. 1981, Braunstein 1982, McGlynn et al. 1982).

The bony architecture of the glenohumeral joint as imaged by CT has been investigated.  In particular, alterations in the glenoid tilt, anteversion angle of the scapula, glenohumeral index and glenoid type have been evaluated.

## MATERIAL AND METHODS

One hundred and sixty-four patients treated for recurrent anterior dislocation of the shoulder over the past ten years at the 1st Department of Orthopaedic Surgery, University of Milano Medical School, Milano, Italy were considered for this study.  The surgical operations carried out were of the Bankart or modified Bristow types and post-surgery follow-up ranged from 3 to 10 years.  The study group consisted of 41 patients (44 shoulders) who were randomly selected from

these patients.   A control group consisted  of  44 individuals selected
from  hospital admission records for primary anterior dislocation of the
shoulder  which  did  not  recur  after  a  five-year  period,  since
redislocations  usually  occurred  within  18  months  (Henry and Genung
1982).

Numerous  previous  reports (McLaughlin and Cavallaro 1950, Rowe  1956,
Hovelius  et al. 1982) have shown age at the time of primary dislocation
to be a very important  factor  influencing  the  prognosis  of  primary
dislocation  of  the  shoulder.    The highest recurrence rate (96%) was
noted among patients under 30 years of age, whereas, in  the  report  by
Henry and Genung (1982) 90% of the 315 non-recurrent cases were over the
age of 30.    Therefore, the age of the patients must be considered  when
evaluating other variables.

The  study  group included 34 males and 7 females, whereas there were
32 males and 12 females in the control group.    No-one in  either  group
was known to have suffered from epilepsy.    The various phases of trauma
in relation to dislocation considered in this study included:

(i)   mechanism of injury (direct blow or indirect violence)

(ii)  fractures (greater tuberosity or anterior glenoid rim)

(iii) nerve injury (axillary nerve)

(iv)  ease or difficulty in reduction.

An inverse relation has been shown to exist between the  violence  of
the  initial  trauma and the incidence of recurrence (Rowe 1956, Rowe et
al. 1978).   Greater external impact on the shoulder would be associated
with  a  lower  recurrence  rate because of the intense repair following
injury.    However, the paired case-control subjects were fairly  matched
(12·3%  and  13·7%)  with  regard  to  relative frequences of the injury
mechanism.

The authors' definition of immobilization considered  only  the  body
bandage, for example, crepe bandage worn for three weeks, as acceptable.
None of the immobilized patients removed the device during this  period.
The  importance  of immobilization for prognosis in shoulder dislocation
is still the subject of much debate (Rowe et al. 1978, Henry and  Genung
1982, Hovelius et al. 1982, Yoneda et al. 1982).

The  Hill-Sachs  lesion  is  difficult  to  define  and identify with
certainty  by  CT.     Strict  criteria  must  be  adhered  to  if
false-positives,  rarely  false-negatives,  are to be kept to a minimum.
A preliminary CT survey in 34 normal subjects revealed in  11  shoulders

flattening of the humeral head which, according to some authors (Rowe 1956, Stoker 1982), constituted a mild defect. Only CT images of a well-defined hatched depression, with or without accompanying sclerosis in the postero-lateral countour of the humeral head, and present only on the affected side were considered acceptable as criteria for diagnosis of Hill-Sachs lesion. Among the study group subjects, 41 (100%) presented with the lesion while it appeared in 37 (84·1%) of the controls. The importance of this lesion in conditioning the recurrence of dislocations is questionable.

Pathological findings have been considered a consequence of the violence of the initial episode and not the cause of recurrence of dislocations; however, DePalma (1973) conceded that some of these abnormalities might facilitate recurrence. They were not considered in this study.

CT scans of the shoulders were carried out in all individuals. On the CT sections that provided adequate visualization of the scapula, glenoid fossa and head of the humerus, measurements for glenoid tilt, anteversion angle of the scapula, glenoid angle, glenohumeral index and glenoid type were obtained. The glenoid tilt ($\delta$), the anteversion angle of the scapula ($\varepsilon$) and the glenoid angle ($\zeta$) form angles of a triangle as shown in Figure 1. The triangle was constructed by tracing a line that joined the glenoid's anterior and posterior bony parts, a line joining the midpoint of the glenoid fossa and the vertebral border and a line running parallel to the horizontal plane.

On the basis of the relationship of the glenoid radius to that of the humeral head, Saha (1981) described three glenoid types:

(i)   type A: glenoid with the radius larger than that of the humeral head;

(ii)  type B: both glenoid and humeral head have the same radius;

(iii) type C: glenoid with a smaller radius than that of the humeral head.

However, in order to carry out statistical testing we obtained the ratio of the radius of the humeral head to the radius of the glenoid.

Considering possible sources of bias, measurements of these angles were determined by each author independently. The mean values of separate angular determinations were then obtained.

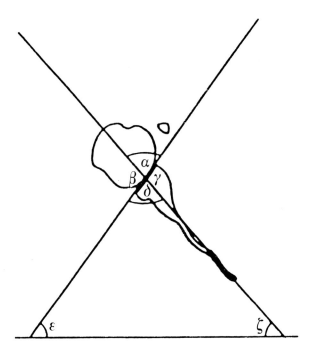

FIG. 1.   Determination of the static parameters:glenoid tilt ($\delta$),
          glenoid angle ($\zeta$), anteversion angle of the scapula ($\varepsilon$).


## RESULTS

The measurements for the glenoid tilt, anteversion angle of the scapula,
glenoid angle, glenohumeral index and glenoid type were obtained for
individuals of both study and control groups.

   A tendency for higher values of glenoid tilt in addition to lower
mean values for anteversion angle, glenoid angle, glenohumeral index and
glenoid type was apparent in the study group as compared to the control
group.   Statistical testing revealed the difference to be significant
when comparing the mean values of the glenoid tilt ($p < .001$) and glenoid
type ($p < .0002$) , while no such difference was revealed for anteversion
angle, glenoid angle and glenohumeral index.      These data are
summarized in Table 1.

Table 1.

Comparison of different parameters in the study group versus the control group.  Figures are Means.

|  | GLENOID TILT | ANTEVERSION ANGLE | GLENOID ANGLE (degrees) | GLENOHUMERAL INDEX | GLENOID TYPE |
|---|---|---|---|---|---|
| STUDY GROUP | 82·3 | 43·8 | 54·0 | 58·9 | 0·73 |
| CONTROL GROUP | 77·4 | 46·9 | 55·9 | 63·7 | 0·95 |
| SIGNIFICANCE | p<.001 | N.S. | N.S. | N.S. | p<.0002 |

## DISCUSSION

Recurrent dislocation of the shoulder does not have a primary or main cause but rather represents the result of multiple factors.  Since determinants of stability are multifactorial, involving both static (structural) and dynamic (muscular) components, instability represents the combination of inherent structural imbalance and the resulting forces expended at the weakest point of the shoulder.

The value for the glenoid angle is a function of two separate indices:  the glenoid tilt and the anteversion angle of the scapula. This relationship exists since they are angles of the triangle whose sum is 180°.  Considering the model shown in Figure 2 – in A, when the anteversion angle is held constant, the glenoid angle varies inversely as the glenoid tilt, i.e. as the glenoid tilt increases or decreases, the glenoid angle decreases or increases respectively.  In B, the glenoid tilt is held constant and the glenoid angle decreases as the anteversion angle increases and vice versa.  It should be realized that in any individual the glenoid tilt is constant, and independent of what its value may be.  The anteversion angle on the other hand is a dynamic measurement, subject to within-individual variations.

The biological importance of the glenoid tilt is readily apparent when one considers the ill-effect it would produce on the anterior capsular mechanism.  It has been shown that no single anatomical structure is responsible for glenohumeral stability at any position of the arm.  Different components come into play with increasing abduction of the arm (Turkel et al. 1981).  It follows that this increased strain, i.e. resisting anterior slipping of the humeral head would be

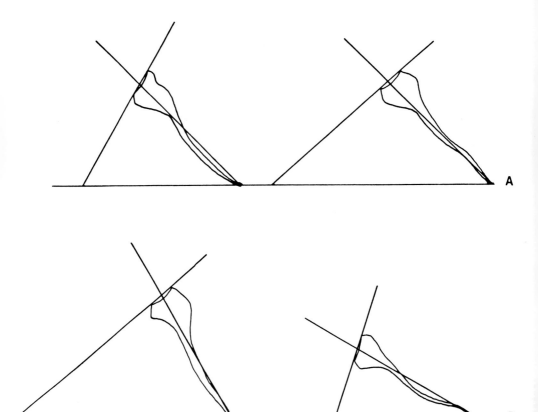

FIG. 2.    Diagram illustrating changes in the glenoid angle as a
function  of  the glenoid tilt (A) and the anteversion angle (B).    In A
the glenoid  angle  will  increase  or  decrease as  the  glenoid  tilt
decreases or increases.    In B the glenoid angle varies inversely as the
anteversion angle changes.

imposed  on  progressively  alternating  structural  components  of  the
anterior capsular mechanism.

    The role of the anteversion angle of  the  scapula  in  promoting  or
contributing to glenohumeral  stability  is  still  uncertain.    Barton
(1982) has reported a few cases of abnormally high values of anteversion
angle  for which an explanation could not always be provided.    However,
he  observed  agenesis  of  the trapezius, a short clavicle and thoracic
deformation as the probable explanation for anteversion  in  his  cases.
In our study the anteversion angle did not appear to correlate well with
the thoracic configuration.    Gross bony deformities were  not  observed
and  could  not  be  assumed  to  explain differences in the anteversion
angle.    However, the anteversion angle seemed to be a function of  the

balance of the axial-scapular muscular activity.   We speculate that   it
represents   a   functional   adjustment   to   improve   stability   in   an
inherently imbalanced shoulder.   In one   of   our   patients,   presenting
with  glenohumeral hypoplasia due to an obstetric brachial plexus injury
it was noticed that despite the normal thoracic configuration and normal
clavicular length, motor paralysis at the shoulder caused a 10° decrease
in the anteversion angle on the affected side.   Therefore, mobility   of
the   scapula   as   assessed   by its anteversion angle may be an important
stabilizing factor of the glenohumeral joint.

    A high anteversion angle would also place a   greater   strain   on   the
anterior   capsular   mechanism   (Figure 3).   The figure illustrates that
external rotation must accompany increases in the anteversion   angle   if
the   forearm   is   to   be   held   in   the   same position facing forwards.
External rotation however would stretch the structural components of the
anterior   capsular mechanism and predispose to premature degeneration of
its tissues.

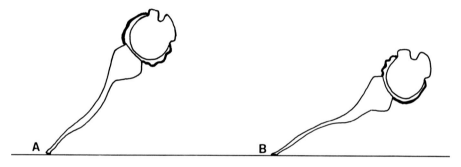

FIG. 3.    Diagram illustrating the   anterior   capsular   mechanism   in   a
shoulder   with   anteversion.     Inevitable   stretching   of   the   capsule
accompanies external rotation of the arm.

    The   glenoid   angle   which is a function of both the glenoid tilt and
the   anteversion angle, due to their trigonometric relationship, was not
significantly   different   (p>.05)   in the two groups unlike the   glenoid
tilt   (p<.001).    This probably is the result of a "functional" decrease
of the   anteversion   angle   in   shoulders   with   a   high   glenoid   tilt.
Therefore   individuals   with   a   high glenoid tilt in conjunction with a
high anteversion angle are more prone to recurrence of dislocation   than
those   subjects   with   a   high   glenoid tilt and reduced anteversion
angle.    In   the   former   unfavourable   situation   one   would   expect   an
abnormally low glenoid angle since their sum must be equal to 180°.

    The   glenohumeral   index   is a function of the contact surface of the humeral head and the glenoid. Normal values never approximated 100%; however high values correlated with increased glenohumeral stability. The lower percentages, though not statistically significant (p>.05), observed among study group subjects may lead towards recurrence of shoulder dislocation.

The glenoid type reflects the shape of the glenoid in relation to that of the humeral head. It considers the effective or actual points of contact of the articular surfaces. It is apparent that a type C glenoid (value more than 1) is the most unstable condition (p<.0002).

Abnormalities of the bony elements of the glenohumeral architecture are not the only factors contributing to recurrence of shoulder dislocation among these patients. Among the forces acting to prevent dislocation are the muscle tone and tension in the enveloping rotator musculo-tendinous cuff; paramount among these is the subscapularis muscle, which promotes glenohumeral stability from 0° to 45° of abduction (Turkel et al. 1981). A similar role is played by the ligamentous components of the anterior capsular mechanism, which alternate among themselves as glenohumeral stabilizers with increasing degrees of abduction.

The algebraic sum of all these factors will dictate the stability of the glenohumeral joint. A functional excess of stability would help the glenohumeral joint to withstand any abnormal forces acting upon it.


## CONCLUSION

Several authors have advocated early surgical repair of recurrent anterior dislocation of the shoulder in the younger age group to slow down the early degenerative changes that may develop (Rowe et al. 1978, Sutro and Sutro 1982).

It is hoped that early recognition of the factors predisposing to recurrent anterior dislocation of the shoulder may aid in planning treatment. Eventually successful management of primary dislocation by immobilization and rehabilition or surgical correction may be based upon the status of the patient's inherent shoulder stability. DePalma (1973) has stated that restoring neuromuscular co-ordination and balance can be achieved only if the bony elements of the joint have a normal or nearly normal configuration.

CT survey may prove helpful in identifying such patients at  risk  of developing  recurrent dislocation of the shoulder and guide in selecting appropriate treatment.


## SUMMARY

A CT study of the bony architecture of the shoulder  in  two  groups  of patients affected with various  types of instability was carried out. The glenoid tilt, glenoid  angle,  anteversion  angle  of  the  scapula, glenohumeral index and glenoid type were the bony parameters compared in the two groups of the study.  The glenoid tilt ($p < .001$)$;$  glenohumeral index  ($p < .0002$)  and  glenoid  type  ($p < .0002$) were the most sensitive indexes in determining shoulder instability.  CT scan of  the  shoulder may be useful in identifying those patients susceptible to recurrence of dislocation and planning treatment.


## REFERENCES

Barton, N. J. (1982).  Anteversion of the  shoulder.   A  rare  clinical sign.   In:   Shoulder Surgery.   (Eds. Bayley, I.  and Kessel, L.). Springer, Berlin, Heidelberg, New York;  pp. 98-100.

Braunstein, E.  M.  and  O'Connor,  G.  (1982).   Double-contrast arthrotomography  of  the  shoulder.  Journal of Bone and Joint Surgery, 64-A:  192-5.

DePalma, A. (Ed.) (1973).  Surgery of the shoulder.  2nd edition.  J. B. Lippincott Co., Philadelphia, Toronto;  pp. 408-417.

Henry,  J. H. and Genung, J. A. (1982).  Natural history of glenohumeral dislocation  revisited.   American  Journal  of  Sports  Medicine,  10: 135-137.

Hovelius,  L.,  Eriksson, K., Fredin, H., Hagberg, G., Weckström, J. and Thorling, J. (1982).  Incidence and prognosis of  shoulder  dislocation: a  preliminary  communication.  In:  Shoulder Surgery.  (Eds. Bayley, I.

and Kessel, L.). Springer, Berlin, Heidelberg, New York; pp. 73-75.

McGlynn, F. J., El-Koury, G. and Albright, J. P. (1982). Arthrotomography of the glenoid labrum in shoulder instability. Journal of Bone and Joint Surgery, 64-A: 506-518.

McLaughlin, H. L. and Cavallaro, W. U. (1950). Primary anterior dislocation of the shoulder. American Journal of Surgery, 80: 615-621.

Rowe, C. R. (1956). Prognosis in dislocation of the shoulder. Journal of Bone and Joint Surgery, 38-A: 957-977.

Rowe, C. R., Patel, D. and Southmayd, W. W. (1978). The Bankart procedure. A long-term end-result study. Journal of Bone and Joint Surgery, 60-A: 1-16.

Saha, A. K. (1981). Recurrent dislocation of the shoulder. 2nd edition. George Thieme V, New York.

Stoker, D. J. (1982). The radiology of the humeral defect in anterior dislocation of the shoulder. In: Shoulder Surgery. (Eds. Bayley, I. and Kessel, L.). Springer, Berlin, Heidelberg, New York; pp. 84-86.

Sutro, C. J. and Sutro, W. (1982). Delayed complications of treated reduced recurrent anterior dislocation of the humeral head in young adults. Bulletin of the Hospital for Joint Diseases, 42: 187-216.

Symeonides, P. P. (1972). The significance of the subscapularis muscle in the pathogenesis of recurrent anterior dislocation of the shoulder. Journal of Bone and Joint Surgery, 54-B: 476-483.

Turkel, S. J., Panio, M. W., Marshall, J. L. and Girgis, F. G. (1981). Stabilizing mechanisms preventing anterior dislocation of the glenohumeral joint. Journal of Bone and Joint Surgery, 63-A: 1208-1217.

Yoneda, B., Welsh, P. and MacIntosh, D. L. (1982). Conservative treatment of shoulder dislocation in young males. In: Shoulder

Surgery.    (Eds.    Bayley,  I.  and  Kessel,  L.).    Springer,  Berlin,
Heidelberg, New York;  pp. 76-79.

## 10. THE EVOLUTION OF THE LIVERPOOL SHOULDER REPLACEMENT

F. H. Beddow
T. R. Redfern

## MARK I PROSTHESIS

In 1969 the need for a prosthetic replacement for the badly damaged rheumatoid gleno-humeral joint became apparent. A constrained cobalt-chrome prosthesis with conventional conformation was designed to fill this need. It was first inserted in 1972. The Mark I prosthesis comprised a 20mm spherical humeral head whose stem was cemented into the humeral shaft. This articulated with a deep metal cup with an attached stem which was inserted into the axillary border of the scapula giving a relatively constrained articulation (Figure 1).

The axillary border of the scapula was chosen because our experience had shown that in rheumatoid arthritis the glenoid could be extensively eroded in its superior and central parts, but the axillary border was always intact and provided a reasonably long cavity for intramedullary stem fixation.

This Mark I shoulder produced excellent relief of pain but the necessary provision of a neck on the head of a constrained prosthesis altered the centre of motion and made the greater tuberosity move through a circle of greater radius. This caused the greater tuberosity to impinge on the acromion and limited the range of movement at 90° of abduction. Four of the Mark I prostheses were inserted. Two patients have subsequently died of unrelated causes and two continue to attend the clinic. Both have rheumatoid arthritis and have painfree shoulders but very little gleno-humeral movement.

## MARK II PROSTHESIS

In 1974 in order to obviate the impingement problem a new prosthesis was
designed with the help of Dr. Martin Elloy of the Department of
Bio-engineering at the University of Liverpool.   In this prosthesis the
ball and socket were reversed, as had been described by Reeves and
colleagues in Leeds in 1972.   A high density polyethylene socket 30mm
in diameter was cemented into the humeral head and a 20mm stemmed
stainless steel sphere was cemented into the scapula (Figure 2).

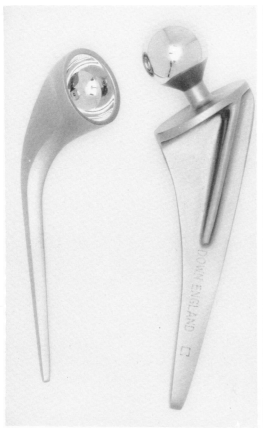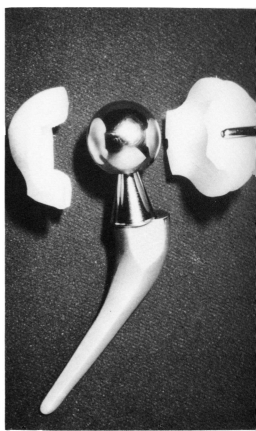

FIG. 1.    The Mark I prosthesis.

FIG. 2.    The Mark II prosthesis ("the Liverpool Shoulder").

The humeral component had a relatively shallow socket to avoid
contact between its rim and the neck of the glenoid component, but   it
extended  beyond  the equator in two places to aid stability and prevent

dislocation until a new fibrous capsule developed. It had a marking wire around its longest equator and a discardable high density polyethylene cap which assisted in the correct alignment of the component so that the lugs did not later cause impingement.

Known as "the Liverpool Shoulder", this design brought the true centre of rotation closer to the anatomical centre of rotation at 25mm from the surface of the glenoid, and overcame the problems of impingement. The axillary border was again chosen for fixing the scapular component but with increasing operative experience it became clear that in rheumatoid arthritis the normal cancellous bone in the upper part of this area was frequently replaced by sclerotic reactive bone, making reaming difficult and fixation less than perfect. A shorter glenoid stem was designed in an attempt to forestall this problem.

At that time it was difficult to obtain sufficient information about the state of the glenoid because conventional radiographs proved inadequate, but recently the advent of the CT scanner has allowed more accurate pre-operative assessment of the scapular bone stock prior to surgery.

Accurate placement of the components is essential for a successful outcome, and a modification of the original Henry approach to the shoulder joint was developed in 1977 to provide wide exposure. The modification involved an osteotomy of the lateral one third of the clavicle, detaching the anterior one third with its attached deltoid unscathed. Reattachment was by simple cerclage and early rehabilitation was possible without fear of detachment of the deltoid from the clavicle. Quite independently, Professor Angus Wallace from Nottingham has adopted the same approach.

This prosthesis was used successfully on 20 patients, 12 prostheses had the conventional stem and 8 had the shorter glenoid stem. All but one patient had excellent relief of their pain but gains in range of movement have been less gratifying, with an average gain of 30° of flexion (range -40 - +80) and 20° of external rotation (range -35 - +70).

Loosening of the scapular component has been a major problem, occurring in 7 of the 20 patients (35%) between 2 and 6 years after operation (mean 3·5 years). This loosening has affected the more active patients but not those who demand little from their prosthetic shoulder due to severe rheumatoid involvement of other upper limb joints.  We believe that our attempts to reproduce the anatomical centre of rotation by mounting the scapular ball 25mm from the glenoid surface, produced a long lever arm which magnified the forces which tended to loosen the scapular component.  Furthermore, constrained joints do not benefit from the cushioning effect of the cuff musculature.

## MARK III PROSTHESIS

Loosening of the scapular component with time and the disappointing gain in movement prompted further research at the University of Liverpool and along with many other centres we now believe that the best option is an unconstrained prosthesis since this causes the least torque at the vulnerable scapular bone-cement interface and the smallest risk of loosening.  The resulting Mark III shoulder is therefore of the unconstrained type.  It consists of a 39 millimetre spherical stainless steel head on a stem which is similar to that of the St. Georg prosthesis.  It articulates with a shallow high density polyethylene saucer originally fixed into the scapula by a short central peg.

Occasionally during total shoulder replacement surgery a patient is seen with an irreparable rotator cuff lesion.  Unless something is done to stabilise the humeral head it is pulled up by the deltoid muscle until it makes contact with the acromion.  This does not necessarily cause pain but is clearly undesirable.  Upward migration of the humeral head is prevented by the insertion of a separate high density polyethylene buffer into the underside of the acromion in patients with irreparable rotator cuff tears.  The large circumference of the humeral component ensures that a congruous articulation between the head and the buffer is maintained throughout the normal range of shoulder movement, so that at no point does the buffer come into contact with the bony humerus.  The buffer permits increased restraint of the humeral component without increasing the torque on the glenoid component and predisposing it to loosening.

Although we have not seen loosening of the glenoid using this unconstrained prosthesis, we are aware that fixation of the glenoid component remains the "Achilles Heel" of total shoulder prostheses and

in 1984 we modified the glenoid component.    This now has two diverging
prongs, one for the axillary border of the scapula and one  towards  the
base  of  the  coracoid process (Figures 3 and 4).    This prosthesis has
been used on 24 patients between July 1980 and July 1986.    Results with
this Mark III prosthesis have  been  encouraging, with every patient
obtaining  good relief of  their  pain.    Gains  in movement  have  been
modest  when  compared  to the results of Dr. Neer, but are in line with
the published results of other U.K. workers.    An  average  20  degrees
gain  in  flexion  (range -20 - +60) and 28° of external rotation (range
-10 - +110) have been achieved.

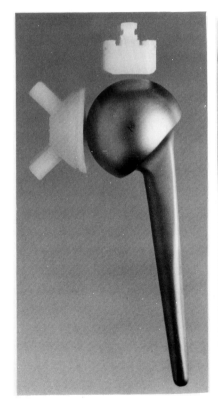 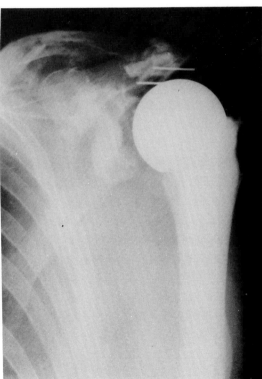

FIG. 3.    The Mark III prosthesis including the buffer.
FIG. 4.    X-ray of a Mark III prosthesis with 3 components.

Research continues at the University of Liverpool into the design and
fixation  of components for total shoulder replacement and into the most
effective rehabilitation regimens  to  maximise  the  benefits  of  such
prosthetic surgery.

## ACKNOWLEDGEMENTS

The  authors wish to thank the Department of Medical Illustration at the
Royal Liverpool Hospital and Ms. Lesley Pratt for preparing the
illustrations.

## REFERENCE

Reeves, B., Jobbins, B., Dowson, D. and Wright, V. (1972). A total
shoulder endoprosthesis. Engineering in Medicine, 6: 64.

# 11. BONE TUMOUR REGISTRIES

## P. D. Byers

The idea of co-operation in the field of bone tumours is not new and is steadily growing. A now traditional vehicle for this is the bone tumour registry, the model for which is that at Bristol, started by Godfrey Price. This is dependent on the enterprise of an individual, but there is inherent in it participation by others through contributing cases and joining in meetings and discussions.

The objective of a bone tumour registry is to contribute to the understanding of bone tumours through:-

(i) epidemiology

(ii) research

(iii) education.

There are obvious limitations to the epidemiology and research that can be carried out, but there is ample scope for education, and through it the registry can make an indirect contribution to patient management.

The traditional registry works retrospectively. An advance on this comes about when the specialists concerned in the management of bone tumours combine forces to provide an advisory service. To some extent every registry does something along these lines in that whoever is running the registry has access to those with expertise in other disciplines, and who can be called on when there is a request for help. But what I have in mind is the arrangement that has been in service at the Royal National Orthopaedic Hospital, London since the mid-sixties whereby the specialists meet as a group on demand to discuss the diagnosis and management of a case. In practice this means that within a few days of a request, and not more than a week, the referring consultant or his representative can present his case to a Panel of experts: surgeon, radiologist, pathologist, biomedical engineer, oncologist and radiotherapist.

This arrangement was established when it became apparent that the traditional method of a surgeon asking for the opinion of surgical colleagues about the management of a case - which resulted in a note in the patient's case records - was an inadequate way to assemble the expertise necessary for good judgement in a difficult case. Even so, it took some years of lively discussion before the members of this advisory group began fully to comprehend one anothers' terminology and expertise. The local success of this group led to making the service more widely available. It gradually expanded to the point of formal recognition by the Department of Health, as a Supra-regional Bone Tumour Service.

There seems good reason why every bone registry should attempt to offer a similar prospective advisory service. There is no doubt in my experience that this is an effective way to improve diagnosis and treatment. It has the added advantage that it brings the case to notice early enough to improve the opportunities for research through increased availability of fresh tissue. This depends upon close co-operation between individual specialists and the registry. This advantage could be compounded through close co-operation between registries. In this way, if regional bone tumour centres covered the country, the basis for sound epidemiological data could be established. The Office of Population Censuses and Surveys is interested in this possibility, and, of course, such relationships do nothing but enhance the educational role of registries.

A scheme of relationships is shown in Figure 1. There are many points in these ideas which could be enlarged upon, and many aspects about which to argue. What progress has been made? There are registries, functioning and potential, to be found throughout the United Kingdom, and generally located in the more densely populated sites. In addition there is a National Bone Tumour Panel, formed in 1960 to serve the first Medical Research Council (MRC) treatment trial; although it no longer serves the MRC it currently accommodates the interests of twelve osteoarticular pathologists. Some of these sit on the MRC Osteosarcoma Working Party and represent the U.K. on the Medical Research Council/European Organization for Research into Treatment of Cancer Pathology Panel. This Panel, has in its turn, started to develop a working contact with the highly organised German speaking tumour groups which cover nine countries; and some tentative steps may

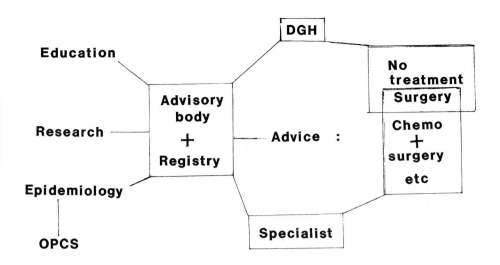

FIG. 1.    The role of a bone tumour panel.

be taken to draw together bone tumour centres in the more Westerly
European countries.    The objectives are the same — to extend
epidemiological data;  to ensure uniformity of criteria, for instance in
diagnosis and in the assessment of the response of osteosarcoma to
chemotherapy;  and to co-ordinate research.    Hopefully, they will come
to realisation.

## 12.INTRA-OPERATIVE BONE SCANNING IN ORTHOPAEDICS

E. P. Szypryt
C. L. Colton
J. G. Hardy

## INTRODUCTION

Radiopharmaceuticals have been used with great success to aid in the detection of occult skeletal neoplasms and infections. A variety of radionuclides have been used for skeletal scintigraphy, technetium 99m labelled methylene diphosphonate (MDP), probably being the commonest in current use. Its high bone uptake, rapid blood clearance and reduced radiation make it ideally suited for medical imaging.

Often clinicians need to obtain biopsies of pathological tissues. Plain radiographs may fail to demonstrate lesions so vividly seen on skeletal scintigrams. Tomographic radiographs and computerised tomography can help in the precise localisation of these lesions preoperatively, but biopsy sites may still be extremely difficult to locate at operation if the external appearance of the bone is normal.

This problem is exemplified during the excision of an often elusive osteoid osteoma. This benign tumour of bone, first described by Jaffe (1935), occurs usually in adolescents or young adults. It can arise in any bone, but most commonly occurs in the long bones of the lower limbs and the axial skeleton. Cortical lesions have the typical appearance of a central lucency corresponding to the nidus surrounded by a zone of sclerosis. However, in cancellous bone, and particularly in juxta-articular lesions, they excite little in the way of a sclerotic reaction and may, therefore, be overlooked on standard radiographs.

Fortunately they almost invariably concentrate radiopharmaceuticals, (Lisbona and Rosenthall 1979, Smith and Gilday 1980). Currently only a single case has been reported of a proven osteoid osteoma with a normal radionuclide bone scan (Fehring and Green 1984).

It is widely accepted that complete excision of the nidus will effect

a cure.   Although occasional recurrences have been recorded it is   not
uncommon   for   patients to   undergo   several   operations   because   of
incomplete resections.   In such difficult cases   excessive amounts   of
healthy tissue may be excised in the search for the all-important nidus.

In   an   attempt   to   eliminate   this   problem the   concept of
intra-operative, scintigraphic bone scanning was   developed.   Accurate
per-operative   localisation   of   these   benign tumours facilitates total
removal of the central nidus, thereby effecting a complete   cure   whilst
avoiding removal of excessive amounts of healthy tissue.

In   1976   a steriliseable probe using a sodium iodide detector with a
fibre-optic link was developed by two of the authors (C. L.   Colton   and
J.   G.   Hardy).   Unfortunately,   several   technical   difficulties were
encountered because of the hygroscopic properties of the   sodium   iodide
crystal   and   optical energy losses within the fibre-optic cable (Colton
and Hardy 1983).   This led to the development of a new probe based on a
cadmium telluride detector system.


## MATERIAL AND METHOD

The   new portable radiation probe is a cadmium telluride crystal mounted
in a collimator, 10mm in diameter with a 3mm window, and attached via   a
14cm   long   handle   to   a cable connected to a compact scaler-ratemeter.
The   equipment   is   manufactured   by   Radiation   Monitoring   Devices,
Massachusetts, U.S.A.

Approximately   three   hours   before   surgery each patient is injected
with a suitable dose of 99m Tc - MDP.   After adequate exposure of   the
bone   the   probe   is   moved   along   its   surface.   The (low) background
readings together with the (high) target readings are recorded so that a
target-to-background   ratio   can   be   calculated.   After removal of the
suspected lesion the resultant cavity is   scanned   to   ensure   that   the
readings have returned to normal background levels.


## RESULTS

Thirty   seven   patients with proven osteoid osteomata have been operated
upon using both probes.   There   were   26   males   and   11   females with a

maximum  incidence  occurring  in the second decade.   All patients have
been followed for a minimum of three months.

Between June 1976 and 1983 the sodium iodide probe  was  used  in  20
patients.   The  majority  of lesions occurred in the long bones of the
lower limbs.   It is worth noting that in only 5 instances (25%) was the
target—to—background  ratio  greater than 2·5.   There were six noteable
failures;  two due to deterioration of the fibre—optic cable;   two  due
to  the  high  background readings causing difficulty in identifying the
lesion and in one case the surgeon thought the probe had been of  little
use  in  reducing  the  amount  of  bone  resection.    In all cases the
immediate  postoperative  recovery  was  satisfactory  but  one  patient
developed  recurrent symptoms probably due to an incomplete resection of
the tumour.

In contrast,  the  cadmium  telluride  probe  has  been  used  in  17
confirmed cases since 1983.   Once again the commonest sites were in the
femur and tibia.   The target—to—background ratios were  always  greater
than  2·5.   There has been no instance of equipment failure but in one
case the surgeon felt it was of little use in  reducing  the  amount  of
dissection,  and  there has been one case of incomplete resection.   Two
further patients developed postoperative discomfort at the site  of  the
original  lesion  but  subsequent  radionuclide  scans have shown only a
diffuse increased uptake.   Surgical  re-exploration  in  one  case  has
failed to demonstrate a residual osteoid osteoma.

In  general the target—to-background ratios were higher when measured
with the cadmium telluride probe than those  obtained  with  the  sodium
iodide  detector.    This  difference  in  sensitivities  is  highly
statistically significant (p<0·001).


## DISCUSSION


Osteoid osteoma has proved an ideal lesion  on  which  to  evaluate  the
technique  of intra-operative bone scanning, since this benign tumour is
often difficult to see on standard radiographs,  but  almost  invariably
concentrates bone-seeking radiopharmaceuticals.

The  probe  has  also  been  used  at  operation to locate other bone
lesions which display a discrete increased uptake of 99m Tc - MDP.   For
example,  to locate metastatic  deposits  for  biopsy,  to  aid  in  the

localisation of small foci of sepsis and to a lesser extent to help differentiate between living and necrotic bone during operations for chronic osteomyelitis. Its greatest advantage is that it will allow accurate localisation of the lesion, ensuring its complete excision without removal of excessive amounts of healthy tissue. The new cadmium telluride probe has proved to be more durable, reliable and sensitive than its earlier counterpart.

## REFERENCES

Colton, C. L. and Hardy J. G. (1983). Evaluation of a sterilizable radiation probe as an aid to the surgical treatment of osteoid osteoma. Journal of Bone and Joint Surgery, 65A: 1019-1022.

Fehring, T. K. and Green, N. E. (1984). Negative radionuclide scan in osteoid osteoma. Clinical Orthopaedics and Related Research, 185: 245-249.

Jaffe, H. L. (1935). Osteoid osteoma: a benign osteoblastic tumour composed of osteoid and atypical bone. Archives of Surgery, 31: 709-728.

Lisbona, R. and Rosenthall, L. (1979). Role of radionuclide imaging in osteoid osteoma. American Journal of Roentgenology, 132: 77-80.

Smith, F. W. and Gilday, D. L. (1980). Scintigraphic appearances of osteoid osteoma. Radiology, 137: 191-195.

## 13.HIP ROTATIONPLASTY FOR MALIGNANT TUMOURS OF THE FEMUR

Winfried W. Winkelmann

## INTRODUCTION

The technique of rotationplasty using the ankle and foot as a replacement for the knee joint is not new. It was first introduced by Borggreve in 1930 for a patient with a shortened lower limb and a stiff knee following tuberculosis. Salzer and colleagues (1981) introduced rotationplasty for the treatment of malignant tumours of the distal femur.

The treatment of choice for malignant tumours of the proximal femur, particularly in patients who are still growing, is disarticulation of the hip or hemipelvectomy. As a surgical alternative in these patients I used the 180° rotated knee joint as a hinge hip joint, the ankle and foot functioning as a knee joint. The details of this technique and the initial results have been published (Winkelmann 1983, 1986).

Three indications for hip rotationplasty have now emerged.

## INDICATIONS FOR HIP ROTATIONPLASTY

### Type I
The indication for a type I hip rotationplasty is in malignant tumours of the proximal femur with maximal proximal extension to the intertrochanteric region, with no involvement of the hip joint and no infiltration of the gluteal muscle (Figure 1).

To give adequate clearance the gluteal muscles can be transsected approximately one inch from their insertion, and the iliopsoas muscle at the point where it emerges through the inguinal ligament. The femoral nerve is also divided at this point. The sciatic nerve has to be

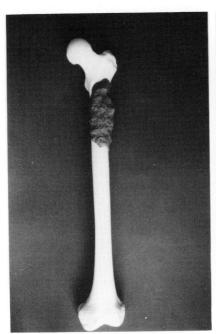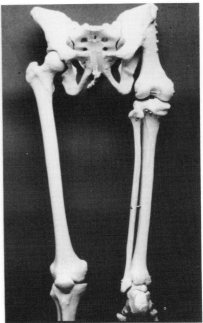

FIG. 1.   Hip rotationplasty type 1.

preserved and dissected distally, whereas the femoral artery and vein
are segmentally resected.    Sufficient distal femur is left so that it
can be fixed to the wing of the ilium with four to five screws.    Active
flexion of the knee joint, now functioning as a hinge hip joint is
effected by the gastrocnemius muscle and the remaining iliopsoas muscle
which is sutured to the hamstring tendons.    Active extension is
effected through the remaining gluteal muscle which is sutured to the
distal tendon-muscle-flap of the quadriceps muscle.

## Type II

The indication for type II hip rotationplasty is in malignant tumours of
the upper part of the proximal femur with involvement of the hip joint
and the surrounding soft tissue (Figure 2).

   In this case a similar operation to the Bank-Colemann-hemipelvectomy
is carried out, leaving part of the wing of the ilium.    The entire
gluteal muscle and the lower part of the iliopsoas muscle are removed,

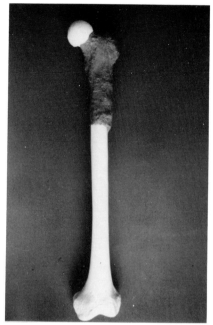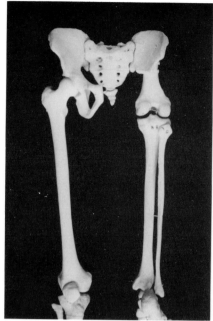

FIG. 2.   Hip rotationplasty type II.

and the femoral artery and vein are segmentally resected.   The  sciatic
nerve  has  to  be  preserved  and dissected distally.   If possible the
branches of the femoral nerve which are distributed into the distal part
of the quadriceps muscle are also dissected distally.   This part of the
quadriceps muscle then functions as an active extensor.   Active flexion
is  mainly  carried  out by the gastrocnemius muscle as often only small
parts of the iliopsoas muscle can be preserved.

Passive movement is comparable to  type  I  but  active  movement  is
distinctly worse.

## Type III

Type  III  is for tumours which require complete resection of the femur.
It can also be applied for distal and proximal tumours of the femur with
skip metastases (Figure 3).

The  sciatic  nerve must be totally dissected out, the femoral artery
and vein are segmentally resected, and the femur  is  disarticulated  at
the  hip  and knee joint.   The tibia is attached to the pelvis with the
help of an endoprosthesis.

Until the distal femur unites to the wing of the ilium patients with type I and type II hip rotationplasty are fitted with a synthetic cast which allows for active exercises. Patients with a type III hip rotationplasty can be immediately fitted with a prosthesis.

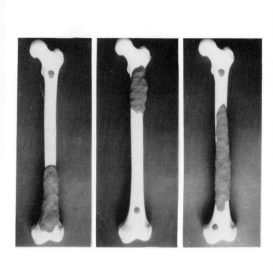 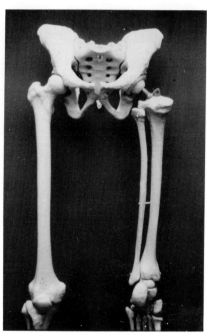

FIG. 3.   Hip rotationplasty type III.


## PROSTHETIC CARE

A provisional prosthesis is fitted within the first postoperative week to support the patient until standard care is possible. This prosthesis is principally of cosmetic value but also allows for active and passive movements of the foot. The shape of the prosthesis is best adapted to that of the contralateral leg. On the lateral proximal end of the prosthesis a pelvic belt is attached over a hinged splint, which gives additional lateral stability of the knee joint for its new function as a hip joint. We prefer the foot embedded in firm synthetic foam.

All of our patients with a rotationplasty are fitted with a

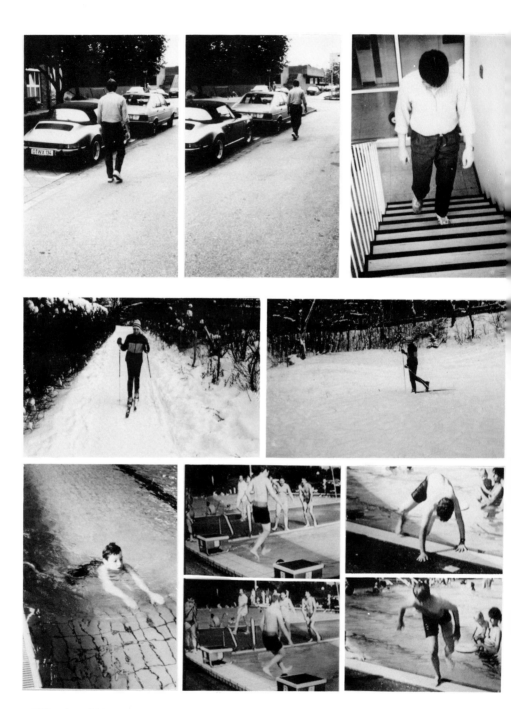

FIG. 4. All patients have a hip rotationplasty.   Shown are some of the
daily activities and sports which are possible.

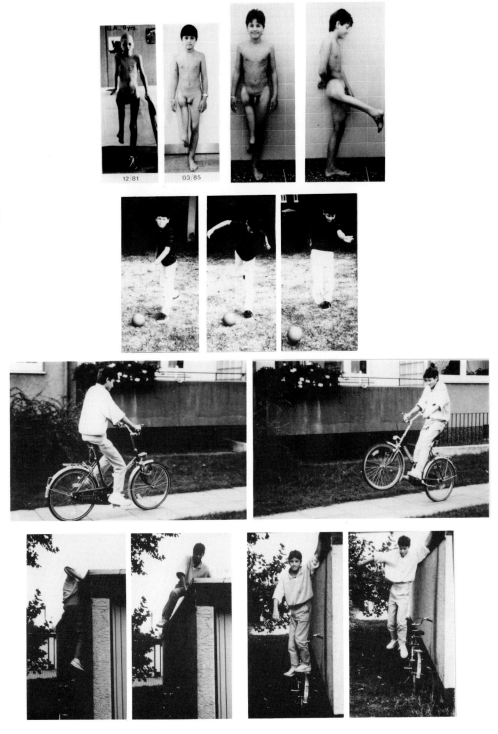

FIG. 4.    Continued.

waterproof swimprosthesis. This is of great importance, as it allows
the patients, who are mostly children, to move about freely in public
swimming pools and to go swimming. The swimprosthesis is adapted for
each individual so that on entering the water it fills up with water
until it reaches the weight of the contralateral leg and thus does not
float. The advantages of a hip rotationplasty, compared with the
handicap following a hip disarticulation or hemipelvectomy is shown in
Figure 4.


## DISCUSSION

In children and young adults with a malignant tumour of the proximal
femur it is important to consider the possibility of a hip
rotationplasty before carrying out a disarticulation of the hip or
hemipelvectomy. Inhibitions arising from the cosmetic disfigurement
can be overcome. Detailed psychological investigations have shown that
all patients with a rotationplasty were happy to have retained a part of
their limb, particularly their foot even when it was rotated. All
patients reported a sensation, thanks to the preserved foot, of standing
with two feet on the ground. The active mobility of the prosthesis,
which functions as a replaced hip and knee joint, is a great advantage.


## REFERENCES

Borggreve, W. (1930). Kniegelenkersatz durch das in der Beinlängsache
um 180° gedrehte Fubgelenk. Arch. Orthop. Unfall-Chir., 28: 175.

Salzer, M., Knahr, K., Kotz, R. and Kristen, H. (1981). Treatment of
osteosarcoma of the distal femur by rotationplasty. Archives of
Orthopaedic and Traumatic Surgery, 99: 313-136.

Winkelmann, W. (1983). Die Umdrehplastik bei malignen proximalen
Femur-tumoren. Zeitschrift fur Orthopadie und ihre Grenzgebiete, 121:
547-549.

Winkelmann, W. (1986). Hip rotationplasty for malignant tumours of the proximal part of the femur.  <u>Journal of Bone and  Joint  Surgery,</u>  68-A: 362-369.

14.
# COMPLICATIONS IN MAJOR PROSTHETIC REPLACEMENT OF LONG BONES FOR TUMOUR AND TUMOUR-LIKE CONDITIONS

J. N. Wilson
J. T. Scales

## INTRODUCTION

Although endoprosthetic devices are known to have been used to repair skull defects as long ago as the time of the Incas, it was not until 1943 that the first major prosthetic replacement for a tumour of a long bone was described. During the next 25 years there were sporadic reports, usually of single cases, indicating that these large implants were satisfactorily tolerated in the human body. Since then a number of centres have taken on the work, which is now recognised as an acceptable procedure, and several large series have been reported. The Department of Biomedical Engineering of the Institute of Orthopaedics, Stanmore, has been in the forefront of the development of new prostheses and over the past 36 years 722 major implants have been supplied to surgical units, mainly in the London and Birmingham areas. Of these, 566 were inserted for the treatment of tumour or tumour-like conditions, the rest being for trauma, failed prosthetic replacement for arthritis, other non-tumour disease of bone or congenital defect. As the technique is becoming widespread throughout the Western World, it was thought opportune to define some of the complications that already have been encountered. The present study is based on a series of 91 operations performed by two surgeons (the late H. Jackson Burrows and J. N. Wilson) using the same operative technique, the same types of prosthesis and the same follow-up management; and in terms of the Enneking classification of local tumour resection these operations could be regarded as a wide excision. In order to achieve this conformity replacements for non-tumorous conditions have been excluded as well as the early prototypes where plastics and side plates were used in manufacture. The patients studied have been confined to replacements of the femur, humerus and tibia using intramedullary stem fixation with polymethylmethacrylate bone cement* introduced by means of a pneumatic cement gun.

## MATERIAL AND PATIENTS

Only the complications which could lead either to prosthetic revision or to amputation have been included in the review, although cases where the prosthetic operation was abandoned in favour of amputation have been added as a failure of the technique. The complications to be considered are listed in Table 1. There were no immediate deaths attributable to the operation, but deaths possibly related to local recurrence have been recorded and these have been compared with the total death rate in the series. The unexpectedly high incidence of local recurrence was disturbing and this has been analysed in detail.

Table 1

Complications occurring in a series of 91 patients

| | |
|---|---|
| Operations abandoned in favour of amputation | 2 |
| Infection | 1 |
| Breakage (includes 1 osteoporotic fracture) | 5 |
| Loosening | 4 |
| Dislocation (hip) | 6 |
| Local recurrence | 18 |

## RESULTS

Operation abandoned

Every patient in this series for whom a major prosthetic replacement was advised first had to agree to the alternative treatment by amputation should the tumour prove unsuitable for replacement. There were,

*Simplex P or C (or a mixture of P and C) polymethylmethacrylate bone cement supplied by Plastics Division, Howmedica International Inc., London.

however, only two such cases.   In one of these, a chondrosarcoma of
femur, the soft tissue mass was much larger and less well defined than
expected before operation, rendering a safe excision impossible; while
in the other, a rapidly growing giant cell tumour of tibia, it was not
possible to excise the tumour without sacrificing a large area of skin
which, in the case of a tibial replacement, meant that it would not have
been possible to cover the prosthesis.

## Infection

The only infection occurred after an initially successful replacement of
the lower femur for parosteal osteosarcoma.   An x-ray six months after
operation showed no evidence of infection and clinically the prosthesis
gave excellent service for five years.   At that time the patient
presented with a septic "arthritis" of the artificial knee joint which
rapidly progressed to a generalised chronic osteomyelitis of the upper
shaft of the femur surrounding the intramedullary stem and later similar
changes occurred in the tibia.   The infecting organism was E.coli, and
it is probably significant that prior to the onset the patient had
complained of a long standing paronychia infection, also due to E.coli.
Although an amputation has been advised, this patient has elected to
retain her prosthesis as the infection is kept under reasonable control
by continuous antibiotic therapy.   There seems little doubt that in
this case the infection was blood-borne and supports the view that
patients with major implants should take prophylactic antibiotics if a
bacteraemia is suspected from some other infected area.

## Breakage

The four breakages all occurred in the intramedullary stems of femoral
replacements and were in the early cases where commercially pure
titanium (T5 - Ti160**) was used in the manufacture of the stem.   In
two patients it was possible to revise the replacement but in the other
two it was not possible to remove the broken stem and an amputation was
performed.   There was one additional case where a pathological fracture
occurred through osteoporotic bone immediately above an intramedullary
stem in the upper femur in a case of giant cell tumour of the knee.
This fracture was explored but no evidence of recurrence was found and
the breakage was attributed to disuse atrophy of bone.   Sound union

**Made by I.M.I. Titanium Limited, Birmingham.

occurred with conservative treatment and the patient still retains her prosthesis 15 years later.

## Loosening
There has been loosening of the stem fixation in three patients and loosening of an acetabular cup in one other case. Two of the stem loosenings occurred in upper humeral replacements where only a very small bone fragment could be retained inferiorly. Despite a somewhat horrific appearance, these particular loosenings gave minimal disability in elbow joint function and both patients elected to retain the appliance. The third loosening was in the distal fixation of a proximal femoral prosthesis. It is interesting to note that there has been no loosening in the stem fixation of any of the replacements of the lower half of the femur where, by necessity, a fixed hinge knee joint was used.

## Dislocation
Dislocation occurred in six of the thirty eight patients who underwent excision of the upper half of the femur with total replacement of the hip joint. These dislocations were all post-operative, usually within the first week. They were easily reduced under a general anaesthetic and, after immobilisation in broomstick plasters for six weeks, there were no further incidents of instability.

## Local recurrence
This was the largest, and by far the most disturbing, complication in the series. There were 18 such cases the details of which are listed in Table 2. The total number of patients treated for each disease is given in brackets. A high rate of local recurrence might have been expected where the replacement was performed for very malignant tumours, but it was surprising to find that the recurrence rate was considerably higher (40%) for the much slower growing chondrosarcoma. The reason for this may lie in the selection of cases and in the effect of pre- and post-operative adjuvant therapy. Because of this high incidence the complication of local recurrence has been examined in more detail.

### Cause of local recurrence
It is suggested that there may be four factors predisposing to local

Table 2

Local recurrence after major prosthetic replacement

| Tumour | Number recurred | Total Number of patients |
|---|---|---|
| Chondrosarcoma | 11 | 27 |
| Osteosarcoma | 3 | 8 |
| Parosteal osteosarcoma | 1 | 9 |
| Fibrosarcoma | 1 | 2 |
| Malignant fibrous histiocytoma | 1 | 4 |
| Giant cell tumour | 1 | 17 |

recurrence, and these seem to be particularly relevant for chondrosarcoma. They are: an ill-chosen case; a patient presenting with a pathological fracture; previous attempts at local excision; and inadequate bone resection.

    i.    The ill-chosen case. Five of the recurrences were possibly attributable to this cause, in particular where the tumour had broken clear of the bone cortex without any obvious line of demarcation.

    ii.    Pathological fracture. Three of the recurrences gave a history of a pathological fracture as the presenting symptom. This was usually accompanied by a sudden increase in size of any soft tissue extension, which resulted in difficulty in defining the tumour margins.

    iii. Previous local excision. There were three patients with recurrence who had undergone an attempt at local curettage of the tumour. In one case of chondrosarcoma of the humerus this was no more than a partial excision through tumour tissue. The inevitable recurrence was treated by prosthetic replacement but there was soft tissue extension within a year, which necessitated a forequarter amputation. A recent paper (Cannon and Dyson, 1986) has suggested that a badly sited biopsy scar that can not be easily excised at the time of prosthetic replacement may be the cause of recurrence. While admitting that this may be true, there was only one patient in

this series where the recurrence could have been attributable
to the biopsy, and in this instance the material obtained
through this incision was reported as negative for malignancy.

iv.  Inadequate resection.  Although there was no example of this
following major replacement, there was one case of low grade
chondrosarcoma of the femoral head and neck, later successfully
replaced with a major implant, that in the first instance had
been inadequately treated by replacement with a femoral head
prosthesis only.  At the revision operation there was evidence
of extension of the tumour along the stem of the original
prosthesis.

Management of local recurrence

With the exception of infection, and the two broken stems which could
not be extracted, local recurrence has been the only complication that
has posed a problem of treatment.  Management took the form of local
excision,    amputation,    adjuvant    therapy    (chemotherapy    and/or
radiotherapy) and palliative treatment.   This   group   had   an   overall
death  rate of 66% (12 patients) compared with 16·5% for the series as a
whole.   Only one patient has survived after local excision, while   five
are  still  alive after radical amputation.   There is little doubt that
the results of attempts at limb preservation after local recurrence   are
poor, and the price of procrastination disastrous.


CONCLUSION


Despite the complications outlined the results achieved in the treatment
of tumours or tumour-like conditions over 21  years  using  custom  made
prostheses indicate that, with proper selection of cases and appropriate
technique, this is an acceptable form of   tumour   management   giving   an
improved quality of life compared with the use of artificial limbs.


REFERENCE


Cannon,  S.R.  and Dyson, P. H. P. (1986).  The relationship of the site
of open biopsy of malignant bone tumours to local   recurrence   following

resection.    Paper    to  British  Orthopaedic  Association,  Edinburgh,
September 1986.

# 15

# BONE ALLOGRAFTS FOR THE RESECTION OF BONE TUMOURS OR FOR TRAUMA OF THE LOWER LIMB

D. Poitout
G. Novakovitch
A. Trifaud

## INTRODUCTION

The use of preserved bone is not a recent technique. The first published case of bone grafting was carried out by Van Mechren in Amsterdam in 1810. Allografts have been used since 1879 when Mac Ewen treated a humeral pseudo-arthrosis with fresh graft taken from an amputation.

Since 1971, in Marseille, we have used fresh allografts and after 1981, deep-frozen grafts with excellent results (Poitout 1986, Poitout and Novakovitch 1986). To date, we have treated 167 patients as follows:-

108 cancellous allografts for osteotomy

12 cancellous allografts for Papineau technique or filling of defects

37 cortico-cancellous allografts for acetabular reconstruction

5 massive osteochondral allografts

2 massive diaphyseal allografts

3 massive metaphyseo-diaphyseal allografts with prosthesis

(1 total femoral replacement)

### Cryopreserved allografts
The advantages of banking bone are evident, mainly because bone bank usually was in the dimensions and quality required. This allowed surgical intervention that otherwise could not be carried out.

Allografts were well incorporated by the host bone. The protein matrix and mineral were antigenic, but deep-freezing reduced the immunological reaction because the histocompatibility antigens situated on the cell membrane were partly impaired by the process ( Takagi and

Urist 1982, Friedlaender 1983, Goldberg et al 1984).

Furthermore, when they were compared, there were no significant differences in the incorporation of autologous or allogenic grafts, apart from that of massive allografts which may have taken an extra 3 to 5 months or longer. Both types of graft were revascularized, the dead bone being replaced by creeping apposition (Friedlaender et al. 1982, Burchardt 1983, Weiland et al 1983, Charpentier 1984, Coutelier et al. 1984).

Many methods of preservation have been described, but deep-freezing seemed to be the best way of storing bone without problems (Tomford et al. 1983).

Since 1981, we have stored  deep-frozen  massive  osteo-cartilaginous grafts  in  liquid  nitrogen (at a temperature of -196°C).  This allowed an indefinite preservation of the bone and the preservation of osteo-cartilaginous cellular vitality (Roy-Camille et al. 1981, Poitout 1985, 1986, Poitout and Novakovitch 1986).


Biomechanical properties

The mechanical resistance of cortical allografts was only 50 to 60% of that of normal bone for up to 8 to 18 months after the graft was inserted and until it was revascularised (Poitout 1985, 1986).

Two to three years were necessary for the bone to return to a normal biomechanical density and resistance.

The biomechanical properties could be impaired by the preservation or the storage process. Deep-freezing seemed to ameliorate the allograft's mechanical resistance which reached 110% to 120% of that of fresh bone.

On the other hand, lyophilisation and massive irradiation (more than 3 megarads) led to less mechanical resistance of the grafts (55% for lyophilisation and 60% to 70% for massive irradiation)(Friedlaender et al. 1982, Burchardt 1983).

## RESULTS

## Types of grafts

### Cancellous grafts:

In 1982 we published a comparative study of 219 free autologous and 71 allografts which showed that the histological, immunological and clinical evolution was very similar.

The time required for consolidation was the same for both groups and successive radiographs showed no differences in their incorporation. Since this study, we have used allografts whenever bone grafting was indicated.

### Cortico-cancellous grafts

These are mostly used to rebuild the acetabulum. Between 1981 and 1985 we have reconstructed 37 hips with graft taken from femoral head or neck. In almost every case a prosthesis was also implanted, being cemented in all but two instances, when a non-cemented arthroplasty was used.

The results were excellent. There were no infections, but one graft collapsed after 12 months (in a patient who had undergone 17 surgical procedures and who required grafting of the entire acetabulum).

### Massive diaphyseal and epiphyseo-metaphyseal grafts:

Massive diaphyseal or epiphyseo-metaphyseal replacements could be used with no particular difficulty. Intra-medullary fixation was one of the most useful methods as it left the muscle close to the graft.

Massive prostheses were sometimes associated with long term mechanical problems. Prostheses could be combined with allografts. The prosthesis avoided the problems of cartilage viability and ligamentous laxity, whereas the allograft offered long term incorporation and rapid muscular reattachment.

In three instances we have used massive prosthetic arthroplasties surrounded by allografts.

### Osteo-cartilaginous grafts:

When feasible it may be better to graft only a thin layer of sub-chondral bone so that chondrocyte nutrition can be obtained from the synovial fluid as well as by epiphyseal neo-vascularization.

If the entire capsule, or most of it including the host's ligaments, could be fixed to the graft, the joint stability was satisfactory.

If articular necrosis occurred only partial replacement of the articular surface by a small prosthesis some years later may be required. Residual laxity may justify the use of a prosthetic ligament or human deep-frozen ligament graft.

If muscles and ligaments had to be removed, as was often the case in tumour surgery, it was better to use an articular prosthesis surrounded by an allograft.

## Complications

Complications linked to the use of allografts have been described by several authors, and set the limits for this type of surgery. In addition to local recurrence of tumour there were several complications which are inherent to this type of surgery (infection, fracture, joint instability, necrosis and lack of consolidation). These complications occurred in 1 to 15% of patients, according to different series.

### Infection

This was the most frequent and the most serious complication as it often led to amputation, the removal of the graft, or if the graft could be preserved, the functional results often were poor. To date we have had 3 cases in 167 procedures, an incidence of 1·8%. We usually use per-operative Betadin as well as local and systemic antibiotics.

### Fracture

These occurred during the period of graft incorporation, and in some instances have been due to inadequate osteosynthesis. They were treated like a normal fracture: with osteosynthesis and autologous bone grafting, and usually healed satisfactorily.

### Joint instability

This complication was rare, accounting for less than 5% of complications despite the problems of fixation of the ligaments and capsule to osteo-cartilaginous grafts.

## Necrosis and arthritis

Although the histological appearance of grafted cartilage was abnormal in almost 80% of the cases, long term results did not indicate the development of arthritis or other changes in the morphology of the joint surface 10 years later.

## Failure of incorporation

This complication was quite rare, although an average of 8 months was required for the incorporation of the ends of the graft. If, after this period, the graft was not consolidated, fresh autologous grafts were added.

## CONCLUSION

Our results, based on 167 operations since 1971 indicated that allografts used to replace large osseous defects were well tolerated and incorporated by the host bone. Our aim was to rebuild the bone partly destroyed by trauma, neoplasm, infection, congenital or degenerative disease. The use of osteo-cartilaginous allogenic grafts helped in achieving this aim.

Deep-freezing allowed the preservation of large pieces of bone, in satisfactory conditions of sterilization. This type of preservation maintained the bone architecture in an optimum biological and biomechanical state. Because the cells had been destroyed, and the bone was incorporated by the host's own cells the immunological reaction was diminished.

Although the bone was totally integrated within some years following the grafting, the functional value of any cartilaginous surface was impaired after a massive osteo-cartilaginous graft. Experimental studies of ligament grafts as well as reconstructive prostheses surrounded by deep-frozen allografts gave encouraging results.

## REFERENCES

Burchardt, H. (1983). The biology of bone graft repair. Clinical Orthopaedics and Related Research, 174: 28-42.

Charpentier, B. (1984). Mécanisme du reject des allogreffes. Presse médicale, 13: 2697-2700.

Coutelier, L., Delloye, C., De Nayer, P. and Vincent, A. (1984). Aspects microradiographiques des allogreffes osseuses chez l'homme. Revue Chirurgicale Orthopédique, 70: 581-588.

Friedlaender, G., Mankin, H. and Kenneth, W. (1982). Osteochondral allografts (biology, banking and clinical applications), Little Brown, Boston/Toronto.

Friedlaender, G. (1983). Immune response to osteochondral allografts. Current knowledge and future directions. Clinical Orthopaedics and Related Research, 174: 58-68.

Goldberg, V. M., Bos, G. D., Heiple, K. G., Zika, J. M. and Powell, A. E. (1984). Improved acceptance of frozen bone allografts in genetically mismatched dogs by immunosuppression. Journal of Bone and Joint Surgery, 66-A: 937-950.

Poitout, D. (1985). Conservation et utilisation de l'os de banque. Cahier d'enseignement de la S.O.F.C.O.T., No. 23, Expansion Scientifique - Paris, pp. 157-177.

Poitout, D. (1986). Greffes utilisées pour reconstruire l'appareil locomoteur, Masson, Paris.

Poitout, D. and Novakovitch, G. (1986). Allogreffes et banque d'os. Encyclopédie médico-chirurgicale, Appareil locomoteur, 14015 A 10, Paris, France, p. 6.

Roy-Camille, R., Laugier, A., Ruyssen, S., Chenal, C., Bisserie, M., Pene, F. and Saillant, G. (1981). Evolution des greffes osseuses cortico-spongieuses et radiothépie. Revue chirurgicale orthopédique, 67: 599-608.

Takagi, K. and Urist, M. R. (1982). The role of bone marrow in bone morphogenetic protein-induced repair of femoral massive diaphyseal defects. Clinical Orthopaedics and Related Research, 171:   224-297.

Tomford, W. W., Doppelt, S., Mankin, H. J. and Friedlaender, G. E. (1983).   1983 bone bank procedures. Clinical Orthopaedics and Related Research, 174:   15-21.

Weiland, A. J., Moore, J. R. and Daniel, R. K. (1983).   Vascularized bone autografts.   Experience with 41 cases. Clinical Orthopaedics and Related Research, 174:   87-95.

16.
# THE TREATMENT OF BONE TUMOURS ACCORDING TO THE ORTHOPAEDIC SCHOOL OF ROME

M. Monteleone
L. Mastidoro
S. Lori
F. Remotti
F. Salimei
U. Tarantino

## INTRODUCTION

In this field the aim of our School is to eradicate the tumour as well as obtain the best functional results. The methods and indications differ greatly, depending on whether the lesion is benign or malignant.

Benign tumours show a well differentiated microscopic pattern, that often resembles the tissue of origin, and in which few or no mitoses are seen. They usually enlarge steadily, but slowly and expansively; are usually encapsulated; and most importantly do not metastatize.

These characteristics often allow the surgical treatment to follow functional principles. Indeed, when the tumour is discovered rather early, and in a site where surgery is possible, the surgeon can completely excise the neoplasm and then reconstruct the part.

With malignant tumours the problem is different, since these lesions endanger the patient's life. Microscopically these tumours lack differentiation and often are so atypical of the tissue of origin that they seem to have nothing to do with it. Mitoses are frequent and atypical. These tumours tend to have an erratic rate of growth, and are invasive but above all every malignant tumour sooner or later metastasizes. Resection of the tumour has to be wider than for a benign lesion, in the hope of excising all malignant tissue with a clear margin. However, the tumour may have already metastasized by the time of surgery. The treatment, therefore, is multi-disciplinary, the oncologist being an essential member of the team. It is the advances in chemotherapy that have enabled the orthopaedic surgeon to obtain encouraging results with non-ablative surgery.

## BENIGN TUMOURS

The aim of surgery is to totally remove the tumour by a procedure that allows preservation or reconstitution of function. The choice of surgical technique varies from simple curettage or marginal excision to wide resection, and depends on the histology of the lesion, its localisation within or extension out of the anatomical compartment of origin, the site of the tumour, and the presence of centres of ossification.

When the tumour arises in a site not critical for function (e.g. diaphysis of a long bone) it is possible to carry out a wide resection without endangering function. In more critical sites (e.g. epiphyses and metaphyses of immature bones with open physes) more conservative surgical techniques are indicated. In many instances additional procedures such as bone grafting or internal fixation are required to obtain a full functional recovery.

We use a particular type of cortico-cancellous bone graft - the "column bone graft" ("innesto a colonna" in Italian) which is composed of a cortico-cancellous rod. The cortical component provides the mechanical strength, whilst the cancellous bone provides the biological stimulus for reossification of the postsurgical cavity (Figure 1).

The cortical component has only a mechanical function and can be separated with a power saw, whereas a chisel must be used to divide the underlying cancellous component, in order to respect the latter's viability. The bony rod has to be placed vertically to provide an effective bearing action. It is important to accurately measure the cavity so that the bone graft can be firmly inserted, becoming a true prop. To correctly carry out this technique, the lesion must be widely exteriorized.

We use the tibial crest or the iliac crest as donor sites for this graft. Occasionally other sites, such as a rib and olecranon, are used. The former is suitable for defects in the short, tubular bones of the hand (e.g. in the treatment of chondromas).

A variant is the "shifting cortico-cancellous bone graft". This technique is utilised when the lesion is near a usual donor site. After curettage or excision, a cortico-cancellous bone rod is obtained using the technique described above and is shifted into the cavity to be filled. Only one incision is required and the operating time is

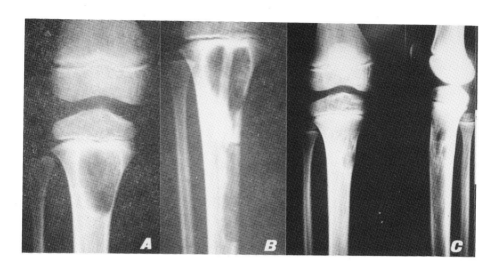

FIG. 1.    a)  Bone cyst in a 4 year old girl;  pre-operative x-ray.
           b)  Post-operative x-ray, "column" bone graft in place.
               The donor site in the tibial diaphysis can be seen.
           c)  Three years after surgery, the lesion has healed.

reduced.

   We prefer the "column bone graft" to bone chips  or  other  types  of
bone  graft, and have some experimental evidence which suggests that the
filling of a cavity with  bone  chips,  causing  an  increase  in  the
intracavitary  pressure  may be an obstacle to osteogenesis ("osteoclast
activation" - Pommer 1919, Lang 1954), and may result in  resorption  of
the bone graft with reformation of the cavity.   Pure cortical rods lack
the cancellous component  that  is  necessary  to  provide  an  adequate
biological  stimulus, whereas pure cancellous grafts lack the mechanical
strength.

   A  pure  cortical  rod  combined  with  cancellous  bone,  even  if
conceptually correct,  may also have major  drawbacks.   First,  the
filling  of  the  cavity  with  the  cancellous  bone  may  increase  the
intracavitary  pressure  and,  as indicated above, lead to resorption of
the graft.   Secondly,  the harvesting of cancellous bone separately from
the  cortical  bone  may damage the cellular component of the trabecular

bone with diminution of the biological stimulus.

If a benign tumour requires a mere radical operation, because of its extension, histological type or age of the patient, a prosthetic replacement is used as indicated below.


## MALIGNANT TUMOURS

The therapeutic problem is more complicated; since these tumours always endanger life, resection must be radical, and treatment is multidisciplinary.

The choice of treatment, the sequence of operations, and the kind and dose of adjuvant therapies depend on many factors. These include the histological characteristics of the tumour, its biological grade, intra-and extra-compartmental extension (Enneking et al. 1980), the prognosis, the responsiveness to adjuvant therapy, the age of the patient, and the patient's psychological profile.

In general, after biopsy, the patient receives one or more courses of combination chemotherapy which may be combined with radiation therapy. We then proceed to surgery, the amount of cellular necrosis in the resected tumour is evaluated and further courses of chemotherapy and/or radiation therapy given. Sometimes, other kinds of adjuvant therapy, such as hyperthermia, arterial perfusion or immunotherapy are employed. We tend to use the newer high-dosage chemotherapeutic regimens.

Because malignant tumours may develop after irradiation, because the results of radiotherapy are not always satisfactory, and as the efficacy of chemotherapy has increased, we have assumed a more critical attitude to the use of radiotherapy. Nevertheless we still use it with clearly responsive tumours such as the Ewing's sarcoma (Marcove and Rosen 1977).

When it is possible to radically but locally resect the tumour, prosthetic replacements are often utilised. In some instances commercially available prostheses are used. For example, with malignant tumours of the distal femur a Shier's type of prosthetic replacement can be inserted, as it preserves the tibia in case arthrodesis of the knee is subsequently required. In other patients, custom-made original prostheses are necessary, but in both instances a modular system is used. Some years ago, we realised that it was impossible to completely programme the surgery for a malignant tumour,

because in many instances the pre-operative evaluation   of  the  tumour
did   not   correspond   to   the   reality seen in the operating room.   The
surgeon must be able to fit the prosthetic replacement into   a   modified
situation   and,   therefore,   our   prostheses   are modular and have rings
which can be inserted round the shaft of the prosthesis (Figure 2).

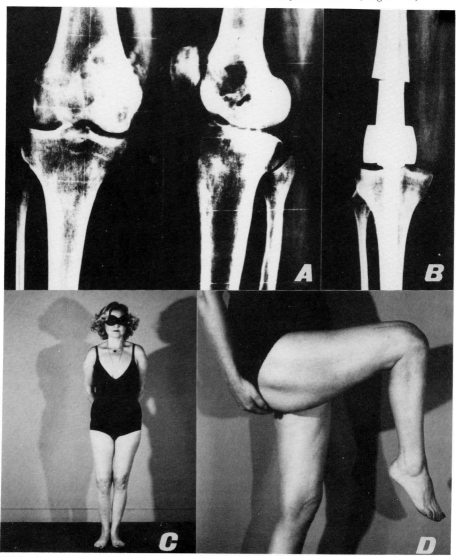

FIG. 2.    a)  Malignant fibrous histiocytoma of distal femur in a 38
               year old woman.   Pre-operative x-ray.
           b)  Post-operative x-ray.   Shiers type prosthesis with
               modular components in place.
           c)  Photograph 2 years after surgery:   aesthetic result.
           d)  Functional result.

Many modular models are now commercially available.

The correct diagnostic and therapeutic approach to malignant bone tumours has to be a team approach, and requires the combined action of surgeons, oncologists, pathologists and radiologists.

The role of the oncologists, radiologists and pathologists is to diagnose, define the prognosis and supervise the medical treatment of the patient, whereas the surgeons' responsibility is to perfect the surgical techniques to obtain radical excision of the tumour but maintain the function of the affected part. When both objects are realised, surgery has attained its aim.

## REFERENCES

Enneking, W. F., Spanier, S. S. and Goodman, M. A. (1980). A system for the surgical staging of musculoskeletal sarcoma. Clinical Orthopaedics and Related Research, 153: 106-120.

Lang, F. J. (1954). Le cisti genuine delle ossa. Arch. Putti, 4: 29.

Marcove, R. C. and Rosen, G. (1977). Ewing's sarcoma functional effects of radiation therapy. Journal of Bone and Joint Surgery, 59-A: 325-331.

Monteleone, M., De Angelis, F. and Papalia, M. (1975). Possibilità chirurgiche in oncologia chirurgica. Atti e memorie della SOTIMI, 31: 51-59.

Pommer, G. (1919). Zur kennitnis der progressiven hämotom und phleghasie veranderungen der rohrenknochen auf grund der mikroskopischen befunde im never knochenzystenfalle. Archiv. Für Ort. und Unfall. Chir., BD 17.

17.
# PATHOLOGICAL FRACTURES OF THE SPINE INCLUDING THOSE CAUSING ANTERIOR SPINAL CORD COMPRESSION:  SURGICAL MANAGEMENT

### M. W. Fidler

## INTRODUCTION

Pathological fracture of the spine, caused by metastases, is one of  the most unpleasant sequelae of malignant disease.  When conservative treatment has been exhausted or  offers  no  hope  of  success,  surgery should be considered.  The indications for operation are:

(i)  Spinal cord, cauda equina or nerve root compression caused by a bone fragment, by tumour which is radioresistant,  or  after  a  maximum dose of radiotherapy has already been given.

(ii)  An  unstable pathological  fracture  which  threatens  the integrity of the spinal cord.

(iii)  Severe pain which persists despite conservative treatment.

Rapidly  growing,  uncontrollable  malignant  disease  is  a contraindication to surgery.

Patients  with  metastases have limited life expectancies.  Any form of surgical treatment should remove or prevent any  compression  of  the neural  structures,  relieve  pain  and  ensure  immediate and permanent stability so that the patients can be  rapidly  mobilised  and  returned home as soon as possible.

There are thus two considerations:  decompression and stabilisation.

### Decompression
Spinal  metastases  usually  occur  in  the  vertebral  bodies and cause anterior spinal cord compression.  The spinal cord is  very  vulnerable to  pressure  and  any  attempt  to remove anterior tumour tissue, via a posterior approach, usually necessitates  cord  retraction  and  further damage.  Thus,  anterior  decompression  is  the logical treatment for anterior spinal cord compression.  The cause of the compression  can be

removed comfortably, safely and under direct vision without, in any way, causing further compression of the dura or the spinal cord.

Laminectomy should only be carried out when the cause of compression is posterior.

## Stabilisation

The various techniques of stabilisation will be referred to subsequently, but basically flexion/compression forces can be optimally resisted by the use of an anterior interbody construction, whereas torsion can be better controlled by a rigid posterior rectangle and cement construction.

## PRE-OPERATIVE INVESTIGATIONS

In addition to the plain radiographs, a skeletal scintigram is useful to demonstrate any unsuspected metastases in neighbouring vertebrae as well as any distant skeletal metastases. The extent of the spinal lesion is further assessed by tomograms.

Myelography, followed by CT, defines the precise zone of neural compression, and MRI probably will become very useful. Prior to anterior surgery in the thoracic and lumbar regions, selective angiography reveals the blood supply of the tumour and is usually followed by tumour embolisation, unless a local medullary feeder artery is present.

## Biopsy

If there is any doubt as to the nature of the lesion, biopsy is essential. A needle is used for the vertebral bodies, but for a posterior lesion open biopsy is safer.

## PATIENTS

This review is based on a personal series of 50 consecutive patients, some of whom have previously been described (Fidler 1985, 1986). Each region of the spine can conveniently be considered separately. As the spinal cord usually extends down to L1, this level has been included with the thoracic spine.

## Cervical Spine

There were 16 patients, in all of whom severe pain persisted, with nerve root compression in 4 patients.   One patient had minor anterior  spinal cord  compression caused by a fracture dislocation of C2 which responded to pre-operative traction.   All patients had an  unstable  pathological fracture with the associated danger of spinal cord compression.

### Decompression

The  involved  roots  were  decompressed  by  removal of the involved laminae and facets.

### Stabilisation

Posterior stabilisation is simple at all levels and has the merit  of effectively providing the rotational stability which is essential in the neck.   Initially, simple posterior stabilisation techniques using wires and  grafts  were  used,  but it soon became obvious that improved rigid posterior fixation could be  achieved  by  wiring  the  laminae  of  two vertebrae above and below the lesion to a contoured, snug-fitting, rigid tent shaped  rectangle,  and  reinforcing  the  construction  with  bone cement.

For  lesions  involving  the  axis,  the  base of the occiput must be included.   An actual rectangle was unsuitable and so  a  special  rigid plate  was designed (Figure 1).   The plate was carefully screwed to the occiput in the midline where the internal occipital crest is  more  than 1cm thick and then wired to the appropriate laminae.

In  patients  with  a poor prognosis, the construction was reinforced with cement on both sides.   If the prognosis was more than six  months, cement was used on one side and healthy cancellous bone autograft on the other.

## Thoracic-L1 spine

There were 24 patients.   Severe  persistent  pain  was  present  in  5 patients,  anterior  cord  compression  alone in 1, and a combination of anterior cord compression and severe pain in 18 patients.

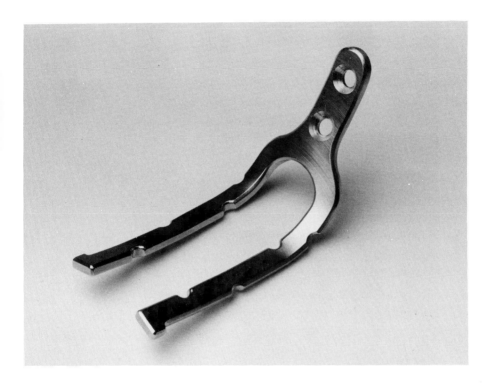

FIG. 1.   The plate for posterior occipito-cervical stabilisation.

### Decompression

An  anterior approach  is  essential  for safe anterior decompression
of the spinal  cord.    The  lesion  was  approached  via an  appropriate
thoracotomy,  except  for  T1,  which  was  approached  via  the    neck.
Following ligation of the vessels supplying the tumour, a tunnel was cut
through the diseased vertebral body which was  then   removed   piecemeal,
until the dura had been completely exposed and decompressed.

### Stabilisation

A simple modular interbody distractor which was easy  to   insert   was
designed.    By   virtue of its central position, it did not angulate   the
spine.    The distractor was so inserted that   the   lips   of   the   plates
fitted   round the anterior edges of the vertebral end-plates (Figure 2).
This   provided   optimal   mechanical   advantage   for   the   correction   of
kyphosis   and   also   supported   the   vertebral   bodies   at   their   strong
peripheries.    The   defect was then filled   with   liquid   bone   cement,

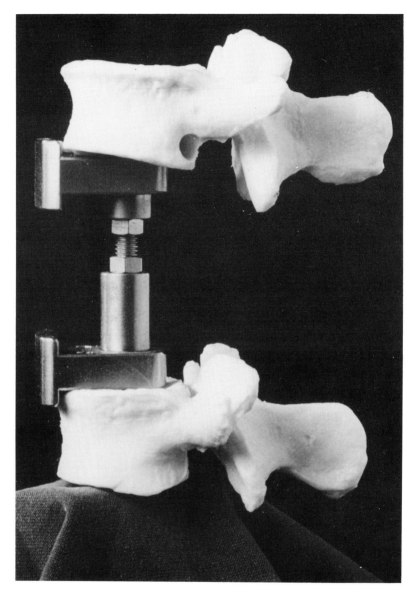

FIG. 2.    A model to show the anterior    interbody    distractor    in    place
following vertebral body excision.

whilst    the  dura  was  protected  by  a  layer  of  gel-foam;    during
polymerisation the area was doused in cold saline.

At  the  thoraco-lumbar  junction,  where  the  rib  cage  does    not
contribute  to stability, the interbody construction was reinforced with
a modified, strengthened paravertebral Zielke system (Figures 3 and 4).

In  3 patients an excellent prognosis was anticipated and a posterior bone graft was added for additional stability.

## Lumbar Spine (L2-L5)

There were 4 patients, 2 of whom complained of unremitting pain, whereas the other 2 suffered from pain combined with cauda equina compression.

Lesions   involving  L2   and   L3   were  treated   by   the   same technique as described  for  the  thoraco-lumbar  junction.    At   L4, anterior stabilisation alone proved inadequate.  Supplementary posterior stabilisation with a rectangle, laminar wires and cement is now added as a  routine  procedure  two weeks later.   Autograft may be preferable to posterior metal and cement if wound healing is felt to be unpredictable, as a result of previous radiotherapy.

In this series there have been no solitary lesions of L5.

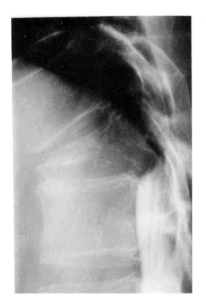 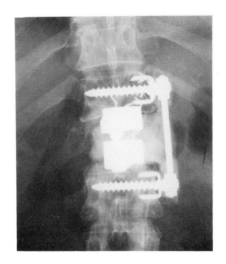

FIGS. 3 and 4.    Pre- and postoperative radiographs.
FIG.  3.    A pathological fracture due to a metastasis in T12 has caused spinal cord compression.
FIG.  4.    The situation following vertebral  body  excision,  spinal decompression and stabilisation.

## Sacrum

So far only one patient with destruction of the first sacral segment has been encountered.  L5 was  also  involved.    The  patient  had  severe persistent low back pain with involvement of the left L5 and S1 nerves.

Following posterior decompression, stabilisation was achieved by means of a sacral bar, two Harrington rods and autograft from the iliac wings to L4.

Posterior instrumentation alone in the thoracic and lumbar regions

Four patients were treated by posterior operations, prior to the development of the anterior technique, and one patient since.

All had severe persistent pain. There also was cauda equina compression in 2 patients, cord compression in one and intercostal neuralgia in one patient.

Laminectomy was carried out in 3 patients. Stabilisation was achieved with Harrington rods and autograft in the first 4, and a rectangle, laminar wires and bone cement in the last patient.

## RESULTS AND COMPLICATIONS

Cervical Spine

Nerve root decompression was effective wherever necessary.

Posterior fusion was successful, but the patients had to remain in traction or wear a brace for up to three months. Posterior instrumentation, reinforced with cement, provided immediate stability and relief of pain in all patients. However tumour progression led to failure of fixation in 2 patients, in one of whom the posterior construction was then extended down to healthy vertebrae. A third patient developed a painful motion segment at the level below the fusion. Anterior interbody fusion relieved the pain.

Thoracic spine + L1

Neurological recovery occurred in 18 of the 19 patients afflicted. The exception died from an "Adult Respiratory Distress Syndrome" without regaining consciousness. One patient with a rapidly growing melanoma developed a recurrence at two weeks after initial recovery and died four weeks later.

Pain was relieved by effective stabilisation, although in one patient with pathological fractures at T8 and 9 and severe osteoporosis, the neighbouring vertebral bodies collapsed over the original type of narrow

rectangular distraction plate five days following operation.   Severe
pain necessitated supplementary posterior stabilisation.    To improve
peripheral load bearing, the plate was modified from the original
rectangular shape to the segment form.    So far this has proved
successful.

## L2 – L5
There was neurological improvement in the 2 patients afflicted.

At L4, anterior stabilisation alone failed in the first 2 patients.
Supplementary posterior instrumentation restored stability.    In the
remaining 2 patients, staged anterior and posterior instrumentation
proved stable, though in one patient, following the passage of a laminar
wire, a CSF fistula developed and thereafter the wound failed to heal.

## Sacrum
Local recurrence led to failure of fixation at six months.   A pressure
sore led to a persistent sinus.

## Posterior approach alone for the thoracic and lumbar regions
There was partial neurological recovery in only one of the 3 patients
subjected to laminectomy.

Pain was relieved satisfactorily in 4 and partially in one patient.

## General Complications
There was excessive bleeding in 2 patients with thoraco-lumbar fractures
prior to the use of embolisation.

There have been no post-operative infections.    Prophylactic
antibiotics were routinely adminstered for 48 hours beginning
half-an-hour pre-operatively.

## Survival
The postoperative survival averaged 10·6 months with a range of 1 week
to 53 months.    The useful survival was shorter due to local recurrence
or, more usually, other metastases and averaged 9·2 months (0 – 53).

As to be expected, the best results were obtained when there was a
surgically correctable mechanical problem in a patient whose disease was
localised and responsive to treatment.    Patients with solitary lesions
lived for 25 months on average, those with a few controllable metastases

13 months, whilst those with multiple metastases survived an average  of only 5 months.


## CONCLUSIONS

When surgery is indicated, the following techniques are applicable.

### Decompression

Anterior spinal cord compression should be treated by anterior decompression. Recovery of an incomplete lesion can be expected. Anterior cauda equina compression should also be decompressed anteriorly.

Posterior decompression for cervical nerve root compression is effective.

### Stabilisation

Cervical spine and T1: posterior instrumentation with a rectangle and cement. Use of the spinal plate (Figure 1) facilitates inclusion of the occiput. Autograft is added when the prognosis is good.

Thoracic spine, T2 to T11: anterior interbody stabilisation.

T12 to L3: anterior interbody stabilisation + paravertebral strengthened Zielke fixation. Posterior autograft may be added when the prognosis seems very good.

L4: combined anterior and posterior stabilisation.

Sacrum: further experience is necessary.

Posterior stabilisation alone in the thoracic and lumbar regions should principally be reserved for the relief of pain in poor risk patients when neural involvement is unlikely, and for the stabilisation of several, non-adjacent painful fractures.

I should like to emphasise that these patients require a multidisciplinary approach with close co-operation between radiologist, radiotherapist, oncologist and surgeon.

ADDENDUM

Since this study was completed, a patient has been referred with a painful pathological fracture of C4 causing progressive anterior cord compression. Anterior decompression and stabilisation restored neurological function and stability.

REFERENCES

Fidler, M. W. (1985). Pathological fractures of the cervical spine. Palliative surgical treatment. Journal of Bone and Joint Surgery, 67-B: 352-357.

Fidler, M. W. (1986). Anterior decompression and stabilisation of metastatic spinal fractures. Journal of Bone and Joint Surgery, 68-B: 83-90.

18.
# INTRAMEDULLARY HYPERTHERMIA IN THE PREVENTION OF PATHOLOGICAL FRACTURES OF LONG BONES DUE TO METASTASES

E. B. MacMahon
B. Sadr

## INTRODUCTION

Pathological fractures of long bones due to metastatic cancer occur with increasing frequency as the survival of cancer patients improves with modern therapy. The orthopaedic surgeon is often asked to stabilise a pathological fracture in a long bone of a patient with advanced disease and a limited life span. In an earlier stage of the disease prophylactic internal fixation of an impending pathological fracture has the advantage of reduced morbidity (Sangeorzan 1986). Clearly it would be better to prevent the occurrence of pathological fractures at a still earlier stage without the need for major surgery.

At present, radiotherapy is the only non-invasive method available for the treatment of skeletal metastases prior to fracture – chemotherapy has a much smaller role. While radiotherapy is often effective in this respect, published data point to an appreciable failure rate – up to 40% in certain radioresistant metastases (Schocker and Brady 1982).

Recently there has been much interest in the use of hyperthermia, which was shown to be effective against mammalian tumour cells (Storm et al. 1979). Its use within the medullary cavity of long bones is interesting in view of the relative tolerance of osseous tissue to heat (Berman et al. 1984).

## MATERIAL AND METHODS

Our experimental model has been the New Zealand white rabbit. VX2 carcinoma injected in the medullary cavity of the rabbit tibia through a drill hole reliably produces fractures at the two metaphyseal ends of bone, which is similar to the site of metastatic fracture often seen in man (Figure 1). Injection of VX2 in both tibiae produces a symmetrical pattern of tumour spread and pathological fracture. One tibia can be treated and the contralateral side can be used as the control.

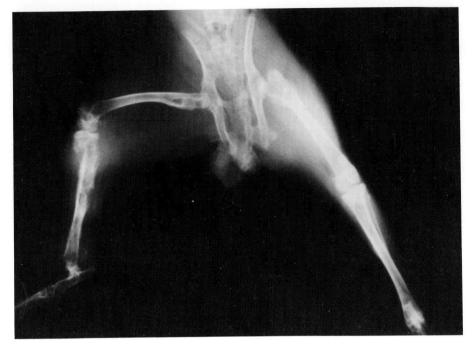

FIG. 1. Pathological fracture of the tibia of a rabbit five weeks after intramedullary injection of VX2 carcinoma.

Having determined the pattern of tumour spread in four rabbits, attention was focused on the effects of intramedullary heating of bone. In two rabbits normal tibiae were subjected to intramedullary heating using a hollow metal tube through which water at 55°C was circulated for 45 minutes (Figure 2). The animals were killed between one and three weeks later, and the tibiae were examined histologically. It was found that heat (55°C) partially destroyed the marrow, but had little effect on the bony envelope in which live osteocytes were still abundant. Furthermore, the surrounding tissue (muscle, fat, skin, etc.) appeared unharmed, apparently protected from thermal injury by the intervening bone.

In a further ten rabbits VX2 carcinoma was injected bilaterally into both tibiae, and at intervals of one week (five rabbits) or two weeks

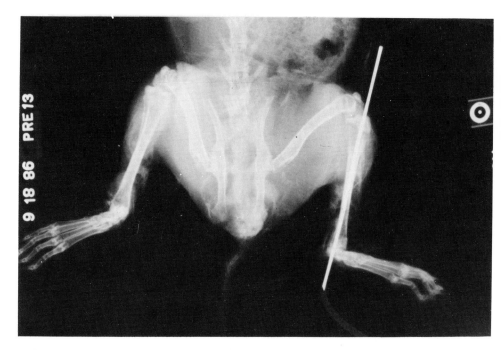

FIG. 2.    Intramedullary heating using a cannula through which water  is circulated at 55°C.

(five  rabbits)  intramedullary  heating was performed on one side only. The animals were subsequently observed, x-rayed at weekly intervals  and killed  upon  the  first  evidence of pathological fracture (usually 3-5 weeks after innoculation with VX2 carcinoma).


RESULTS


Suppression of tumour growth was consistently achieved by intramedullary heating  (Figure  3).   A  pathological  fracture first occurred in the untreated tibia, the treated tibia  becoming  involved  later  and  more slowly.   The  fact  that  hyperthermia  was only able to delay and not totally abolish tumour spread indicated that some tumour cells  survived possibly  due  to  uneven  heating  of  the  tumour mass.   Histological examination revealed necrotic tumour and  marrow  cells  in  the  heated specimens  surrounded by a normal bony envelope in which live osteocytes were abundant.

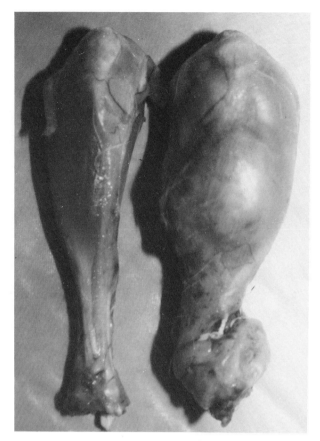

FIG. 3.    Autopsy specimens showing the unheated leg (right side) with obvious tumour involvement and the heated side where the  tumour  growth has been suppressed.


## CONCLUSION


The    data    so    far    indicates    that    there    is    a    definite    role    for intramedullary hyperthermia in the treatment and prevention of  skeletal metastases.     The    thermotolerance    of    bone    makes    it an ideal tissue within which heat can be used for tumourcidal  purposes,  with  relative impunity  and  with  little danger of damage to the surrounding bone and muscle envelope.   The local necrosis of  marrow  is  an  expected  side effect  of this treatment, but not sufficiently important to prevent the use of this technique.

Improvements   in   the   method   of   heat   delivery are currently being studied. Various heating systems, such as interstitial microwave (Lyons et al. 1984), radiofrequency (Sugaar and LeVeen 1979), and ultrasound (LeVeen et al. 1976, Marmor et al. 1979), have been effective in the treatment of various malignancies and appear applicable to intramedullary hyperthermia.


ACKNOWLEGEMENT

This work was made possible by the dedication and co-operation of the Bio-engineering Department of the Veterans Administration, Medical Center, Washington, D.C.


REFERENCES

Berman, A. T., Reid, J. S., Yanicko, D. R., Sih, G. C. and Zimmerman, M. R. (1984). Thermally induced bone necrosis in rabbits. Clinical Orthopaedics and Related Research, 186: 284-292.

LeVeen, H. H., Wapnick, S., Piccone, V., Falk, G. and Ahmed, N. (1976). Tumour eradication by radiofrequency therapy. Responses in 21 patients. Journal of the American Medical Association, 235: 2198-2200.

Lyons, B. E., Britt, R. H. and Strohbehn, J. W. (1984). Localized hyperthermia in the treatment of malignant brain tumours using an interstitial microwave antenna array. IEEE Transactions on Biomedical Engineering, 31: 53-62.

Marmor, J. B., Pounds, D., Postic, T. B. and Hahn, G. M. (1979). Treatment of superficial human neoplasms by local hyperthermia induced by ultrasound. Cancer, 43: 188-197.

Sangeorzan, B. J., Rayn, J. R. and Salciccioli, G. G. (1986). Prophylactic femoral stabilization with the Zickel nail by closed technique. Journal of Bone and Joint Surgery, 68-A: 991-999.

Schocker, J. D. and Brady, L. W. (1982). Radiation therapy for bone metastasis. <u>Clinical Orthopaedics and Related Research,</u> 169:   38-43.


Storm,   F. K., Harrison, W. H., Elliott, R. S. and Morton, D. L. (1979).
Normal tissue and solid tumour effects of hyperthermia in animal   models
and clinical trials. <u>Cancer Research,</u> 39:   2245-2251.


Sugaar,   S   and   LeVeen   H.   H.   (1979).   A histopathologic study on the
effects of radiofrequency thermotherapy   on   malignant   tumours   of   the
lung. <u>Cancer,</u> 43:   767-783.

## 19.OSTEOGENESIS IMPERFECTA:  DIAGNOSTIC CONSIDERATIONS

### P. Beighton

## INTRODUCTION

Osteogenesis imperfecta (OI) is a common and well known inherited disorder of connective tissue. More than 300 affected persons have been studied in Southern Africa (Beighton et al. 1983, Beighton and Versfeld 1985), and it has become apparent that certain diagnostic issues have important implications in orthopaedic surgery. These problems are discussed in this article.

## EVALUATION OF DIAGNOSTIC CRITERIA

### Scleral blueness
In the classical form of OI, blueness of the sclerae represents a major diagnostic criterion. The scleral colour, however, may range from white to a delicate blue tinge, to a slatey grey, making evaluation difficult. There is considerable overlap with normality, especially in infants and persons with dark brown eyes.

The scleral blueness in OI is age-related and sclerae which are sky blue in childhood may become dark grey in old age. Ethnic pigmentation is also important and the sclerae are grey rather than blue in persons with dark skins. It is also possible that scleral colour may fluctuate; some affected individuals have asserted that their scleral colour and tendency to fracture are inter-related. To date these claims remain unsubstantiated.

### Wormian bones
Wormian bones are regarded as pathognomic of OI. These bones are

present in the cranial sutures; they are numerous and have irregular margins, resembling pieces of a jigsaw puzzle. Wormian bones are conventionally visualised in the occipital sutures in lateral skull radiographs, but in difficult cases, a Townes view, taken through the foramen magnum may be very helpful.

Wormian bones are also a component of several rare conditions, such as cleido-cranial dysostosis and the Hadju-Cheney syndrome. They occasionally are a normal variant in the newborn. The most frequent problem in interpretation derives from a rotated skull radiograph, as the resultant overlap of sutures produces an appearance which closely resembles that of Wormian bones.

## Skeletal configuration

In the severely affected person with OI, the skeleton is gracile and porotic with disturbance of growth and deformity consequent upon repeated fracturing. The skeleton may also be malleable, resulting in bowing of the long bones, biconcavity of the vertebrae and temporal bulging of the skull.

It must be emphasized that these changes are very variable. In a mildly affected person with OI the radiographic appearance of the skeleton may be entirely normal apart from the presence of Wormian bones.

## Dental features

Dentinogenesis imperfecta (DI), which presumably is a reflection of the underlying abnormality of connective tissue, is a frequent component of OI. Affected teeth have a pearly grey or purple-brown colour and they are prone to caries and attrition.

It has been proposed that DI is valuable in the delineation of various subtypes of OI. However, although DI can often be deemed to be definitely present or absent, assessment is sometimes a very difficult matter. The author has encountered many affected persons in whom "doubtful" DI has defied specialist dental appraisal and where histological or electron microscopical evaluation has been necessary for accurate diagnosis. The situation is further complicated by the fact that DI may involve the primary but not the secondary dentition, or vice versa, and that some teeth may be involved while others are spared. From the foregoing, it can be concluded that DI is of limited diagnostic significance in the subcategorisation of OI.


## DIFFERENTIAL DIAGNOSIS

### Normality

The question as to whether or not an infant has OI may be raised  by  an untoward  fracture or by the presence of the common dominantly inherited form of this condition in a parent.  This may be a difficult problem as the  sclerae are often blue in normal infants, while the skeleton may be radiographically normal in OI.  The presence of Wormian bones is by far the  most  important  diagnostic  indicator,  but  ambiguity  may arise. Studies of  biological  material  at  the  molecular  level  may permit resolution  of this problem in difficult cases, although this technology is not yet fully established.


### Battered Babies

Multiple fractures in childhood may lead to suspicion of  non-accidental injury,  and  the diagnostic dilemma of OI versus a battered baby is not infrequent.   This important problem has immense legal and  sociological implications and the difficulties are compounded by the fact that OI and battering are not necessarily mutually exclusive.

   The correct diagnosis of trauma may be indicated by features such  as subperiosteal haemorrhage and metaphyseal avulsion.  The recognition of external bruising may also be relevant, although it is  noteworthy  that persons with  OI  sometimes have a bruising tendency.  The presence or absence of Wormian bones  is  probably  the  most  important  factor  in resolving this dilemma.


### Juvenile Osteoporosis

Juvenile  osteoporosis  is a rare disorder which has been the subject of long standing debate and controversy.  Characteristically, the skeleton becomes  porotic  before  puberty,  with  resolution in early adulthood. Fractures and deformity  may  occur  during  the  active  phase  of  the disorder.  The diagnosis is established by the biochemical exclusion of metabolic bone disease and the absence of the classical stigmata of  OI. This  negative  approach  poses  the  question  as  to  whether juvenile osteoporosis  really  exists  as  an  autonomous  syndromic  entity.

Convincing    cases    are    very    few    indeed,    and    this    matter    remains
unresolved.

## Overlap syndromes

Occasional    patients    are    encountered    in    whom    stigmata    of    OI    are
associated with features of other inherited connective tissue disorders.
For instance, blue sclerae and bone fragility have been observed in
conjunction   with a Marfanoid habitus while Wormian bones and a tendency
to   fracture   have   been   documented   in   a   family   with   articular
hypermobility  and dermal extensibility, suggestive of the Ehlers-Danlos
syndrome.    Examples of similar combinations can be   recognised   in   the
literature.

There is little doubt that the majority of these "variants" of OI are
syndromes which have remained ill-defined by virtue of their rarity,   or
lack   of   clearcut   phenotypic   features.    In   view   of   the   size and
complexity of the   collagen   molecule,   there   is   great   potential   for
derangement,   and it is perhaps surprising that "intermediate" disorders
of this type do not present more frequently.


## HETEROGENEITY


It   has long been apparent that OI is heterogeneous and a classification
based   upon   clinical,   genetic   and   radiographic   parameters   was
promulgated   by Sillence   and his colleagues in 1979.    This system had
the advantage of distinguishing the common autosomal dominant form (type
I),   which   is comparatively   mild,   the   infantile   potentially   lethal
form    (type   II)   (Spranger   et   al.   1982)   and   the   rare   autosomal
recessive,   severe   form   (type   III)   (Horan   and   Beighton   1975,
Sillence   et   al.   1986).    Prognostication   and   management   are
facilitated if the patient can be confidently   assigned   to   a   specific
category,   but   this   is not always possible.    In orthopaedic practice,
retention of the older conventional subgrouping   of   the   congenita   and
tarda forms of OI has proved to be of value (Shapiro 1985).

The   limits of syndromic resolution by conventional methods have been
reached;   sporadic, unclassifiable patients are   frequently   encountered
and   it   is   probable   that   there is considerable further heterogeneity
(Sillence 1981, Wynne-Davies and Gormley 1981).    These issues   probably

will be resolved by molecular technology.


## CONCLUSIONS

Although the diagnostic criteria for OI are well defined, in practice, appraisal is not always an easy matter. The nature and frequency of orthopaedic complications differ in the various forms of OI and when medicinal therapy becomes available it is likely that there will be some degree of therapeutic specificity. The molecular basis of the collagen defects which underly OI are currently being elucidated and it is likely that increased understanding of the pathogenesis will improve treatment.


## REFERENCES

Beighton, P., Spranger, J. and Versfeld, G. A. (1983). Skeletal complications in osteogenesis imperfecta: A review of 153 South African patients. South African Medical Journal, 64: 565-568.

Beighton, P. and Versfeld, G. A. (1985). On the paradoxically high relative prevalence of osteogenesis imperfecta type III in the black population of South Africa. Clinical Genetics, 27: 398-401.

Horan, F. and Beighton, P. (1975). Autosomal recessive inheritance of osteogenesis imperfecta. Clinical Genetics, 8: 107-111.

Shapiro, F. (1985). Consequences of an osteogenesis imperfecta diagnosis for survival and ambulation. Journal of Pediatric Orthopaedics, 5: 456-462.

Sillence, D. (1981). Osteogenesis imperfecta: An expanding panorama of variants. Clinical Orthopaedics and Related Research, 159: 11-25.

Sillence, D. O., Barlow, K. K., Cole, W. G., Dietrich, S., Garber, A. P. and Rimoin, D. L. (1986). Osteogenesis imperfecta type III. Delineation of the phenotype with reference to genetic heterogeneity. American Journal of Medical Genetics, 23: 821-832.

Sillence, D. O., Senn, A. and Danks, D. M. (1979). Genetic heterogeneity in osteogenesis imperfecta. Journal of Medical Genetics, 16: 101-116.

Spranger, J., Cremin, B. and Beighton, P. (1982). Osteogenesis imperfecta congenita: Features and prognosis of a heterogeneous condition. Pediatric Radiology, 12: 21-27.

Versfeld, G. A., Beighton, P. H., Katz, K. and Solomon, A. (1985). Costovertebral anomalies in osteogenesis imperfecta. Journal of Bone and Joint Surgery, 67-B: 602-604.

Wynne-Davies, R. and Gormley, J. (1981). Clinical and genetic patterns in osteogenesis imperfecta. Clinical Orthopaedics and Related Research, 159: 26-35.

## ACKNOWLEDGEMENTS

My research was supported by the South African Medical Research Council, the Mauerberger Foundation, the Harry Crossley Foundation and the University of Cape Town Staff Research Fund.

# 20

# OVERHEAD DIVARICATION TRACTION IN THE TREATMENT OF CONGENITAL DISLOCATION OF THE HIP

D. M. Heilbronner
J. R. Gage
J. M. Carey

## INTRODUCTION

There are two factors which must be considered in the treatment of congenital dislocation of the hip (CDH). First, avascular necrosis is not found in untreated hip dislocations and, therefore, is an iatrogenic situation; and secondly, premanipulative traction may decrease the incidence of avascular necrosis. The reported incidence of avascular necrosis has varied greatly ranging from Esteve's report of 69% without premanipulative traction (Esteve 1960) to claims of 0% with traction and abduction prior to manipulation.

In 1963, overhead divarication traction (OHDT) was first used at Newington (Connecticut) Children's Hospital in the treatment of CDH. At the time, many other forms of premanipulative traction were utilized, including well leg spica, longitudinal skin, and skeletal traction. The purpose of this study was to review our use of OHDT and the results over a 20 year period, with particular reference to the incidence of avascular necrosis.

## PATIENTS AND METHODS

The method of overhead traction involved the application of skin traction, utilizing the technique of the senior author (J.M.C.). This involved the meticulous application of the traction as follows:

(i)   Tincture of Benzoin was applied to the skin.

(ii)  The malleoli were well padded with multiple layers of cast padding.

(iii) Beginning distally, a layer of elastoplast was applied circumferentially to the skin.

(iv)  Traction straps were applied to the elastoplast with care
      being taken that the straps did not directly touch the skin at
      any point, particularly in the proximal thigh.

(v)   A layer of webril cast padding was then applied over the entire
      leg, firmly and circumferentially to help diffuse the pressure
      forces from the straps.

(vi)  Roller gauze was rolled over this to reinforce the webril and
      prevent its shredding.

(vii) A traction block was used to keep the straps separated so they
      did not rub against the foot.

Certain precautions were necessary to avoid complications. The most
important was to maintain the knee flexed approximately 15° during
application of the elastoplast and the traction straps. Using this
technique, there have been no neurovascular complications to date. It
also was important to ensure that the moleskin straps were not in direct
contact with the skin as blistering would occur. However, this
blistering cleared rapidly upon trimming of the strap.

The patient was then put into traction with the legs straight
overhead. On approximately the third day, after initial muscle
relaxation had begun, divarication was slowly started. Palpation of
the adductor tendons was the guideline for divarication. As the
adductors stretched, the abduction was gradually increased, and was
never rushed. The amount of weight applied varied from patient to
patient and was dependent upon the child's size. Enough was added to
hold the buttocks just off the bed and allow the lower trunk to act as a
counter weight. The applied weight was monitored frequently and
increased with increasing divarication. The average was 1·1 kg., and
ranged from 0·2 to 2·7 kg.

The traction was maintained at all times and the legs were not
routinely unwrapped. There were no major skin problems, other than the
blistering noted in a few children, and which cleared rapidly upon
trimming the straps.

An advantage to the parents and nurses of this form of traction was
that the child could be removed from the bed, while the traction was
maintained for holding or feeding. The traction was continued for $2\frac{1}{2}$
to 3 weeks, and the divarication gradually increased to 60° of abduction
for each hip as the adductors stretched.

The charts of patients seen at Newington Children's Hospital with a CDH during the past 20 years were reviewed. Patients with myelodysplasia, cerebral palsy, arthrogryposis, or other teratologic forms of hip dislocation were excluded, leaving 388 charts for review.

Since the focus of this study was to determine the incidence of avascular necrosis, associated with overhead divarication traction, the following patients were excluded; those who were not treated in traction, who were treated with other forms of traction, who had less than one year of post reduction follow-up, and who had undergone primary open reduction. This left 110 patients who had been treated in overhead divarication traction available for detailed review.

Newington is primarily a tertiary referral centre, and many patients have had preliminary treatment elsewhere prior to referral. Therefore, two subgroups were formed. Those patients who had received treatment prior to referral were designated Group I (26 patients), and those whose initial treatment was at Newington Group II (84 patients).

## RESULTS

There were 26 patients in Group I, 24 female and 2 male. Twenty-five were caucasian and 1 hispanic. The left hip was involved in 10, the right in 7 and both in 9 patients, 35 hips being affected in the 26 patients. The average age at diagnosis was 8 weeks, and the average age when they were first seen at Newington was 23 weeks. The interval between diagnosis and treatment, and referral to Newington averaged 16 weeks. The types of prior treatment were numerous and varied, with some patients having several methods applied. Upon referral to Newington, the treatment regimen was instituted as described.

The children were placed in OHDT for an average of 18·6 days (range 9-35 days), the shorter period occurring in the early years of the treatment programme (1963-1965). Following traction, all 26 patients had closed reductions carried out. Twenty-five were placed in a spica cast and 1 in a Pavlik harness. The spica was maintained for an average of 18·6 weeks (range 8-36 weeks). Following this, 24 patients were maintained in an abduction splint for an average of 22 weeks full time. Four of these patients were subsequently splinted at night for an average of 26 weeks (range 12-52 weeks).

Seven hips in 6 patients in this group showed changes of avascular necrosis, an incidence of 23% of patients and 20% of hips.

In Group II (those patients whose initial treatment was performed at Newington) there were 74 girls and 10 boys. Seventy-seven were caucasian, 5 hispanic and 2 black. The age at diagnosis averaged 22·5 weeks. The left hip was involved in 48, the right in 24 and both in 12 patients.

Upon admission to Newington, OHDT was begun and maintained an average of 17·5 days (range 5-28 days) with the shorter period again occurring in the 1963-1965 period. Following traction, closed reductions were carried out, and 81 patients were placed in a hip spica and 3 in orthoses. The spica was maintained on average for 17 weeks, after which the 81 patients were placed in orthoses for an average of 5 months full time (range 1-13 months). Thirty-two patients underwent night bracing for an additional 5 months.

The age at follow-up averaged 6 years 8 months and the average length of follow-up was 5 years 11 months. The most recent follow-up in this group of 84 patients was remarkable in that there were only 3 patients who demonstrated changes of avascular necrosis. Two of the patients were among the first treated by this method in 1963 and were maintained in traction for only 5 days and 7 days respectively; and following reduction were placed in frog hip spicas. The third patient was treated in traction for 27 days in 1965, and was held in a frog plaster for $8\frac{1}{2}$ months. In this group with 96 dysplastic hips, avascular changes occurred in 3·1% of hips and 3·5% of patients.

Seventy-seven patients were treated after 1965, when the treatment programme became more firmly established. No changes of avascular necrosis have been noted in these patients initially treated in overhead divarication traction.

## DISCUSSION

One of the most important purposes of the divarication was to increase the area of the "safe zone of Ramsey". Two factors influenced our use of overhead positioning. First, Nicholson and co-authors (1954) found a decrease in vascular filling when the hips were maintained in an extended position, due to compression of the medial circumflex vessel in the psoas pectineal interval.    Secondly, Trueta and others (Trueta 1957, Salter and Field 1960, Salter et al. 1969) have shown that by tightening the hip capsule in the extended position, in a joint whose early adapted position was flexion, major compression of the epiphyseal vessels occurred.

Our results have shown the OHDT is safe and we recommend the use of overhead divarication traction in the treatment of congenital dislocation of the hips for the following reasons:

 (i)   It avoids treating the hip in an extended position in age
        groups where there is a physiologic flexion contracture.

 (ii)  It applies traction on the hip joint in the position it
        occupied in utero, making reduction easier to obtain and less
        traumatic.

 (iii) It allows ease of nursing care and increased parent/infant
        contact and interaction.

 (iv)  The incidence of avascular necrosis is extremely low, and in
        those patients in whom it has been the initial treatment, the
        incidence to date has been zero.

## REFERENCES

Allen, R. P. (1962).   Ischemic necrosis following treatment of hip dysplasia.  Journal of the American Medical Association, 180:  497–499.

Crego, C. H. (1939).  The use of skeletal traction as a preliminary procedure in the treatment of early congenital dislocation of the hip. Journal of Bone and Joint Surgery, 21-A:  353–372.

Esteve, R. (1960).  Congenital dislocation of the hip:  A review and assessment of results of treatment with special reference to frame reduction as compared with manipulative reduction.  Journal of Bone and Joint Surgery, 42-B:  253–263.

Nicholson, J. T., Kopell, H. P. and Mattei, F. A. (1954).  Regional stress angiography of the hip. A preliminary report.  Journal of Bone and Joint Surgery, 36-A:  503–510.

Ogden, J. A. (1974). Changing patterns of proximal femoral vascularity. Journal of Bone and Joint Surgery, 56-A: 941-950.

Salter, R. B. and Field, P. (1960). The effects of continuous compression on living articular cartilage. An experimental investigation. Journal of Bone and Joint Surgery, 42-A: 31-49.

Salter, R. B., Kostuik, J. and Dallas, S. (1969). Avascular necrosis of the femoral head as a complication of treatment for congenital dislocation of the hip in young children: A clinical and experimental investigation. Canadian Journal of Surgery, 12: 44-61.

Scott, J. C. (1953). Frame reduction in congenital dislocation of the hip. Journal of Bone and Joint Surgery, 35-B: 372-374.

Trueta, J. (1957). The normal vascular anatomy of the human femoral head during growth. Journal of Bone and Joint Surgery, 39-B: 358-394.

21.
# CDH AND AVASCULAR NECROSIS. WHAT IS THE OPTIMUM AGE TO PERFORM AN ANTERIOR OPEN REDUCTION?

E. R. S. Ross
D. J. Ford
G. A. Evans

## INTRODUCTION

A review of children presenting late with congenital dislocation of the hip has been undertaken. These children were all treated by Mr. Rowland Hughes, at the Robert Jones and Agnes Hunt Hospital, Oswestry, thus providing an opportunity to study a group with consistent management.

## PATIENTS AND METHODS.

The treatment consisted of preliminary traction, in extension and abduction, followed by examination under anaesthesia and arthrography. An open reduction was performed only if an acceptable medial position of the head could not be achieved by closed reduction. The approach for open reduction was through a standard anterior route, reflecting rectus femoris distally and opening the capsule by a 'T' shaped incision. No additional bony procedure was undertaken with the initial reduction.

The incidence and severity of avascular necrosis (AVN) was established (Kalamchi and MacEwen 1980) in relation to the following variables:

(i)   Chronological age at the time of reduction.

(ii)  Ossific development of the capital epiphysis.

(iii) Integrity of the ligamentum teres (at open reduction).

(iv)  Closed or open reduction.

One hundred and eighty four children were treated.

## RESULTS

### Open reduction

One hundred and fifty children underwent open reduction, of which 11
were bilateral, giving a total of 161 hips studied. The age range was
3 months to 6 years 7 months. The overall incidence of AVN was 13·7%.
When the more severe grades (II, III, IV) only were considered, the
incidence was 8·7%. In addition, 13% of the hips had a transient
granular appearance of the epiphysis, which did not form a dense infarct
or transient flattening. This appearance was not regarded as proven
AVN and was allocated as type 1(a) - the Kalamchi group one being called
1(b).

Ossific development of the femoral capital epiphysis was present in
less than half the under 12 month age group, in the majority of the
13–18 month age group and almost all the over 18 month age group.

In children under 12 months with ossification, almost all had a
normal outcome - one having mild AVN and 1 severe AVN. Whereas, where
ossification had not yet occurred, more than one half developed AVN,
usually of a severe grade.

All children aged 13–18 months with ossification of the femoral head
had a normal outcome, whereas nearly half of the hips without
ossification developed severe AVN.

Children over 18 months with ossification usually had a normal
outcome, and if AVN developed it was mainly mild. When ossification
had not yet developed, just under half the patients had a normal
outcome, in all the others the AVN was severe.

The presence of an intact or spontaneously ruptured ligamentum teres
(10 cases) had no effect on the incidence of AVN, neither did excision
of the ligamentum (58 cases).

The numbers in each group are too small for statistical analysis, but
clear trends are evident. When all the radiographic changes from 1(a)
- IV were considered as an abnormal outcome, the numbers were greater in
each group, and it was possible to statistically analyse the data. The
results indicate that the likelihood of a severe outcome is minimised by
waiting for ossification to occur prior to undertaking surgery.

### Closed reduction

Thirty-four children had a closed reduction, of which 12 were bilateral, giving a total of 46 hips studied.  the age range was 2 months to 5 years.    There were 7 children under 1 year of age and all had a normal outcome.    Children over 1 year were less likely to have a normal outcome.    The overall incidence of AVN was 68%.    This included 21% with questionable AVN of Grade I(a), and 34% with Grade I(b) changes. Fourteen of these 16 hips required secondary femoral or acetabular surgery.    Severe AVN (Grades II, III and IV) occurred in 10·8%.

Only 5 of the hips had an unossified capital nucleus when treated and the data is inadequate to comment on its prognostic significance for closed reduction.

## CONCLUSION

When treating CDH surgically, with the technique described, there would appear to be a window of relative safety against AVN between the ages of 13 and 18 months.    This window can be extended to below 12 months, provided the capital nucleus has started to ossify.    The lack of continuity of the ligamentum teres, or its excision as part of the open reduction, did not increase the incidence of AVN.    In contrast, closed reduction over the age of 12 months was associated with avascular necrosis.

Many factors contribute to the development of avascular necrosis, including possibly the technique of traction (see Page 116).    The method of traction was identical in all patients, whether treated by closed or open reduction, and it would seem reasonable to expect its potential adverse influence to have affected both treatment groups. However, the relatively high incidence of AVN following closed reduction and the totally normal outcome after open reduction, in children aged 12-18 months, with ossified femoral heads, suggests that the traction was not a significant factor.

## REFERENCE

Kalamchi, A. and MacEwen, D. (1980). The incidence and severity of avascular necrosis (AVN). Journal of Bone and Joint Surgery, 62-A: 876-888.

## 22.REASONABLE MANAGEMENT OF CONGENITAL CLUB FOOT DEFORMITIES

### N. J. Blockey

### INTRODUCTION

Early surgery for severe congenital talipes equino-varus has received great emphasis in recent years. These ideas seem to be replacing the older more traditional techniques of manipulation and splintage where surgery was reserved for an age when the pathological tissues were more easily identified.

The dangers of early corrective surgery, i.e. within the first 3 months of life, comprise difficulty in getting a bloodless field, difficulty in identifying the structures to be cut or lengthened, the near impossibility of holding such a tiny foot in plaster until an age when weight-bearing begins and excessive post-operative medial scarring that on occasions worsens the problem. Whilst early medial release should be available in recognised centres in order to compare its long term results with more conservative treatment, its complications may well be too severe for routine use.

### PREVIOUS TREATMENT REGIMEN

In 1966 we published the results of treatment of 186 children with structural congenital talipes equino-varus deformities (Blockey and Smith 1966). Early, repeated, vigorous manipulation was used to correct all elements of the deformity by passive stretching. Denis Browne splintage was used to maintain the correction achieved. This programme continued for the first year when outer raise shoes were fitted to the walking child. In the second year 50% of the feet relapsed into equino-varus. These were treated by radical soft tissue correction through an angled medial incision. If this failed to reproduce a satisfactory plantigrade foot, an outer wedge tarsectomy was performed at around 4 years of age. Five year follow-up showed that 87% had a reasonable result. Their feet were painless and fitted into normal shoes, but many had calf wasting and feet of different sizes with restricted hind foot movement.

## CURRENT REGIMEN

The following criteria, present either at birth or evident within 3 months, were associated with a poor result: males, gross calf muscle wasting, a very deep medial plantar groove, tight skin, and the absence of any depression above the calcaneum posteriorly (Figure I). The most important prognostic factor was the failure to achieve hind foot correction within 6-8 weeks despite vigorous repeated manipulations. Although these feet could be pushed into eversion the skeletal anatomy was not returned to normal and they all required surgical division of the tight collagenous tissues and elongation of the tendons of tibialis posterior and tendo-Achilles.

The policy which then evolved was to treat every affected foot with strong early manipulations since stretching of the tight ligamentous tissues was considered safer than surgery at this age. After repeated manipulation for 6 weeks a decision was made on clinical grounds as to the progress achieved. X-rays were not used. If the equinus was not corrected a posterior release was carried out dividing the posterior ankle and subtaloid joint capsules and lengthening the tendo-Achilles under direct vision. A short 2 mm. diameter Steinmann's pin was then placed transversely through the calcaneum and after the skin was closed a plaster of Paris cast was applied holding the foot in eversion and with downward pressure on the pin to enlarge the angle between tibia and calcaneum. This transfixion pin and plaster cast was the only way we could satisfactorily open up the back of the ankle and subtaloid joints (Figure 2). After 6 weeks the pin was removed and manipulation continued weekly up to one year. Relapse at or about one year of age was again treated by radical postero-medial release concentrating on dividing the collagenous tissue running from the medial malleolus to the navicular in order to allow the navicular to be swung laterally onto the head of the talus. Outer wedge tarsectomy was carried out at around

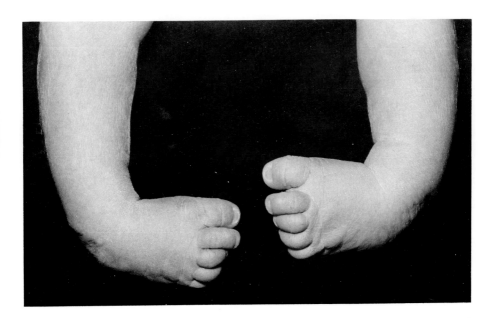

FIG. I.    Clinical appearance of severe club foot.

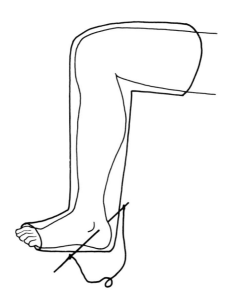

FIG. 2.    Transfixion pin and plaster of Paris cast maintaining hindfoot correction.

the age of 4 in those feet where adduction and midfoot inversion caused tripping and callosities.

Follow-up of children treated in this way showed that 85% were satisfactory in later childhood. There were no instances of ischaemia. None were athletes but none were significantly disabled.

The aim of this regimen was to offer a safe programme shown to produce a foot with which the patient could lead a useful life. Ischaemia, gross shortening due to epiphyseal growth damage, post-operative scarring and other major complications may be caused by too ambitious surgery. We must offer these unfortunate children safe programmes with predictable results.

## REFERENCE

Blockey, N. J. and Smith, M. G. H. (1966). The treatment of congenital club foot. Journal of Bone and Joint Surgery, 48-B: 660-665.

# 23

# TREATMENT OF CONGENITAL PSEUDARTHROSIS WITH ENDOMEDULLARY NAILING AND LOW FREQUENCY PULSING ELECTROMAGNETIC FIELDS (PEMFs): A CONTROLLED STUDY

G. Poli
A. Dal Monte
E. Verni
R. Cadossi

## INTRODUCTION

Congenital pseudarthrosis is an uncommon segmental dysplasia affecting in most cases the tibia at its distal third. This site shows a marked tendency towards pathological fracture, no likelihood of spontaneous healing and high resistance to standard treatment (Codivilla 1907, Camurati 1930).

Characteristic morpho-structural alterations are sometimes already evident at birth or they may appear during the first few postnatal months. The lower third of the leg develops an anterolateral or, occasionally, an anteromedial curvature; and radiographs show sclerosis of the medullary canal or a cystic lesion, shaft shrinkage and associated lesions of the fibula. This corresponds with the pre-injury stage.

A pathological fracture tends to occur at this dysplastic site, and is recalcitrant to any treatment. Even when bone union is achieved, it is short-lived and the pseudarthrosis recurs after some time. The osteogenetic activity is so reduced that it is impossible to maintain an adequate bone structure.

However, the older the patient, the better the response to treatment. It is generally accepted that after puberty the tendency to non-union diminishes.

Therefore, treatment is primarily directed at assuring the longest possible stability of the fracture site, so as to reach puberty. Secondly, treatment is also aimed at promoting the recovery of the osteogenic potential, so that at puberty bone lengthening procedures may be successfully undertaken.

Our experience suggests that immobilization and alignment of the

fracture  site  with  an  intramedullary  nail  (Charnley  1956)  is
satisfactory.    Intramedullary nailing with a Rush nail, inserted  in  a
cranio-caudal  direction,  until  the  tarsus  is  pierced,  allows good
stabilization of the small distal fragment.    In this position the  Rush
nail  inhibits  angular  stresses  and promotes longitudinal compressive
ones.    The same is  not  achieved  with  Boyd's  "double  onlay  graft"
technique (Boyd 1941).    We have used this method in the past and almost
abandoned it in 1975 because of the inadequate mechanical  stability  of
the  distal bone segment and the maintenance of the osteolytic potential
at the site of the lesion.

The results of  grafting,  vascularized  or  otherwise,  cortical  or
cancellous,  autografts or allografts have been poor:  in our experience
they all undergo complete resorption.    There also are drawbacks to  the
fibular  vascularized graft.    There are few reported cases with a short
follow-up and its drawbacks can be summarized as follows.    First, there
can  be  complications  in  the  donor  limb;    secondly, the mechanical
problem is not resolved in that there is insufficient  stabilization  of
the  area;    thirdly,  and  most importantly, the dysplastic site is not
affected by the operation but  the  perichondrial  ring  at  the  distal
tibial physis may be damaged by the surgical procedure.

Thus,  although  orthopaedic  surgeons  can  resolve  the  mechanical
problem, the question of stimulating significant osteogenic activity  to
preserve the osseous structure of the tibia still remains.

Based  on the initial results of the effect of electromagnetic fields
on cell cultures and animals, in 1981 we began to couple  osteosynthesis
by intramedullary nailing with PEMF stimulation of the lower half of the
tibia, including the pseudarthrosis.    This paper is based on our   early
results.


## PATIENTS AND METHODS

Patients  with  congenital pseudarthrosis of the tibia  were enrolled in
the study and randomly subdivided into two groups:  PEMF stimulated  and
controls.    Patients  in  both  groups  were operated upon  by  the
same  team  of  surgeons  with  a  similar  technique:  excision of  the
pseudarthrosis,  reduction  and  alignment  of  the  fracture,  and
osteosynthesis  with  a  Rush  intramedullary   nail  introduced  in   a

cranio-caudal direction from just distal to the proximal metaphysis of the tibia through the subtalar joint. Post-operatively, the limb was immobilized in the identical manner in all patients, namely, a long leg cast for the first 30 days, a walking short leg cast for the subsequent 60 days, and then a leg brace with raises as required for any imbalance. X-rays were taken at monthly intervals for the first 3 months and then at 6 monthly intervals. PEMF stimulation was carried out with a device (IGEA stimulator) delivering an induced electric field of $3 \cdot 5 \pm 1$ mV and generating $1 \cdot 3$ millisecond pulses at a rate of 75 Hz. It began on the third post-operative day and was performed 10 hours daily, not necessarily without a break, but for minimum periods of 1 hour, over 12 months.

## RESULTS

Clinical and radiographic evidence of bone union was not reliable in evaluating the results, because they did not prove to be accurate indicators of long-term union. Therefore, we also used shortening of the limb, compared with the healthy contralateral side and the loss of stability of the nail to assess the results. This loss of stability was shown by bending and breakage of the nail, resulting in further operations to stabilise the tibia. The third criterion determining the treatment quality was the number of operations required.

The results are shown in Tables I and 2. There were no nail "accidents" in the stimulated patients, compared with the controls, presumably reflecting stronger bone in the stimulated patients. Within the 30 month period of follow-up, 3 control patients (50%) developed nail breakage or bending and required further surgery.

Furthermore, during this period, the "length loss" was more marked among control patients than among stimulated ones.

## DISCUSSION

Although some of our patients have been followed for longer, we chose a 30 month follow-up because the nail migrated from the talus within this period and further surgery was required to implant a longer nail.

## TABLE I

### CONGENITAL PSEUDARTHROSIS OF THE TIBIA

Control patients

| PATIENT NUMBER | AGE* (years) | TYPE** | FOLLOW UP | LEG–LENGTH IMBALANCE | NAIL*** | RE–OPERATED |
|---|---|---|---|---|---|---|
| 1 | 1 | 4 | 30 months | Stopped | Yes | Yes |
| 2 | 2 | 3 | " | Stopped | No | No |
| 3 | 8 | 2 | " | Increased | No | No |
| 4 | 8 | 2 | " | Increased | Yes | Yes |
| 5 | 8 | 2 | " | Increased | Yes | Yes |
| 6 | 12 | 4 | " | Increased | No | No |

  * Age of patients enrolled in the study
 ** Classification according to Boyd (1941)
*** Nail bent or broken

## TABLE 2

### CONGENITAL PSEUDARTHROSIS OF THE TIBIA

Stimulated patients

| PATIENT NUMBER | AGE* (years) | TYPE** | FOLLOW UP | LEG–LENGTH IMBALANCE | NAIL*** | RE–OPERATED |
|---|---|---|---|---|---|---|
| 1 | 6 | 2 | 30 months | Increased | No | No |
| 2 | 2 | 3 | " | Stopped | No | No |
| 3 | 4 | 3 | " | Stopped | No | No |
| 4 | 13 | 4 | " | Stopped | No | No |
| 5 | 5 | 3 | " | Stopped | No | No |
| 6 | 5 | 2 | " | Stopped | No | No |

  * Age of patients enrolled in the study
 ** Classification according to Boyd (1941)
*** Nail bent or broken.

These operations, however, were not the same as those to replace bent or broken nails, since they demonstrated that the tibia was growing and losing little or no length compared with the healthy contralateral one.

The enhanced nail stability in the stimulated group assured fewer surgical procedures and hence reduced the risk of iatrogenic damage; skin loss, significant loss of bone or muscle, or infection. Congenital pseudarthrosis often results in amputation. This occurs even in Italy, where, unlike Anglo-Saxon countries, amputation is very seldom accepted by the patient.

Sofield (1971) suggested "keeping by trying", and to follow this advice it is essential to minimise the number of operations. Our study demonstrated that surgical treatment coupled with PEMF electromagnetic stimulation gave better results than surgery alone. Our data, resulting from a controlled study, confirmed those reported by other authors (Bassett et al. 1981, Sedel et al. 1981, Sutcliffe and Goldberg 1982, Sharrard 1984).

A larger number of patients is required to confirm these results. However, at present, PEMF stimulation combined with surgical stabilization with intramedullary nailing of the tibia must be regarded as the method of choice in the treatment of congenital pseudarthrosis of the tibia.

## REFERENCES

Bassett, C. A. L., Caulo, N and Kort, J. (1981). Congenital pseudarthrosis of the tibia: treatment with pulsing electromagnetic fields. Clinical Orthopaedics and Related Research, 154: 136–149.

Boyd, H. B. (1941). Congenital pseudarthrosis: treatment by dual bone graft. Journal of Bone and Joint Surgery, 23: 497–515.

Camurati, M. (1930). Le pseudartrosi congenite della tibia. Chirurgia Degli Organi Di Movimento, 151: 1–162.

Charnley J. (1956). Congenital pseudarthrosis of the tibia treated by the intramedullary nail. Journal of Bone and Joint Surgery, 38-A: 283–290.

134        TREATMENT OF CONGENITAL PSEUDARTHROSIS

Codivilla, A. (1907). Sulle cure della pseudartrosi congenita della tibia. Archivio Di Ortopedia E Reumatologia, 24: 215-232.

Poli, G., Dal Monte, A. and Cosco, F. (1985). Treatment of congenital pseudarthrosis with endomedullary nail and low frequency pulsing electromagnetic fields: a controlled study. Journal of Bioelectricity, 4: 195-209.

Sedel, L., Christel, P., Duriez, J., Duriez, R., Evrard, J., Ficat, C., Cauchoix, J. and Witvoet, J. (1981). Resultats de la stimulation par champ électromagnétique de la consolidation des pseudarthroses. Revue De Chirurgie Orthopedique Et Reparatrice De L'Appareil Moteur, 67: 11-23.

Sharrard, W. J. W. (1984). Treatment of congenital and infantile pseudarthrosis of the tibia with pulsing electromagnetic fields. Orthopaedic Clinics of North America, 15: 143-162.

Sofield, H. A. (1971). Congenital pseudarthrosis of the tibia. Clinical Orthopaedics and Related Research, 76: 33-42.

Sutcliffe, M. L. and Goldberg, A. A. J. (1982). The treatment of congenital pseudarthrosis of the tibia with pulsing electromagnetic fields: A survey of 51 cases. Clinical Orthopaedics and Related Research, 166: 45-47.

# 24

SURGICAL TREATMENT OF THE CHILD WITH DUCHENNE MUSCULAR DYSTROPHY (DMD)


J. D. Hsu


## INTRODUCTION

During the past two decades, many significant changes have been made in the care of the child with Duchenne Muscular Dystrophy (DMD). Active treatment has replaced palliative care, resulting in increasing longevity in a more comfortable environment. The overall management of the DMD child has changed significantly because of studies contributed from leading neuromuscular centres around the world (Endo 1969, Roy and Gibson 1970, Pirot 1972, Siegel 1972, Spencer 1973, Falewski de Leon 1977, Gardner-Medwin 1979, Shapiro and Bresnan 1982, Williams et al. 1984, Seeger et al. 1985, Galasko 1986, Hsu 1986). There is emphasis on prolonging ambulation, the avoidance of fixed contractures and the maintenance of function. The purpose of this study was to review the surgical methods used in the present care of these severely physically disabled children, whose progressive course of muscle weakness leads them to live abbreviated lives with early loss of independence and function.


## PATIENTS AND METHODS

Ambulatory patients:
At Rancho Los Amigos Medical Center, 24 patients with positively diagnosed DMD and their families were introduced to a programme whose goal was to prolong ambulation. Treatment was offered to DMD patients who had reached an age and phase when walking became laboured. They were unsteady, fell frequently (Sutherland et al. 1981), and were becoming dependent on a wheelchair.

The following procedures were carried out.

(i)     Equinovarus contractures of the ankle and foot were corrected by percutaneous tendo-Achilles lengthening (TAL) and posterior tibial tendon transfer anteriorly through the interosseous membrane (PTT) (Hsu 1976) and the iliotibial band was released at the knees if contractures were present.

(ii)    Following the surgical procedure, the limbs were immobilized in long leg casts for 5-6 weeks.

(iii)   The casting was followed by the use of bilateral long leg braces (KAFO).

Post-operatively training was provided by our Physical Therapy Department, as well as on an out-patient basis if needed when the braces were applied. The children were encouraged to walk unaided and were reviewed in the clinic at three monthly intervals. If any problems arose, they were seen at the next clinic or on an emergency basis. The 24 children were followed until ambulation ceased. Other DMD children whose parents elected not to participate in the surgical phase of the study were also followed and served as "controls" for this study.

Wheelchair dependent patients:

A second study was carried out on a further 40 DMD patients. They were older, wheelchair dependent with progressively collapsing spines despite supportive treatment in the form of containment-type body jackets (TLSO), specially fitted seating, or the use of seating support systems (Gibson et al. 1975, Carlson and Winter 1978, Hsu 1983, Rideau et al. 1984, Young et al. 1984). Spinal fusion was carried out when the spinal collapse became progressive and uncontrollable, especially when the patient's arms were used to support the trunk, limiting upper extremity function and table-top activities (Sakai et al. 1977, Siegel 1982, Swank et al. 1982).

RESULTS

Ambulatory patients:

The age at which the surgical procedures were carried out ranged from 8 years to 12 years 5 months. The average age was 10·0 years, a time when muscular dystrophy children were expected to be non-ambulatory and

wheelchair dependent.   All of the children walked for over one year
after surgery, 22 were walking at the end of the 2nd year and 17 of the
24 patients were walking at the end of the 3rd year.   The age when the
children ceased walking ranged from 9 years 9 months to 16 years 11
months with an average age of 13·3 years.

All the patients showed progressive and increasing weakness.   This
was the main reason why they ceased walking and was due to the
progressive nature of the disease in 23 of the 24 patients.   Other
factors contributing to the progressive difficulty in standing and
walking included the development of knee flexion contractures in 8
patients; increase in body weight in 3 patients; fractures of the
lower limb in 2 patients and psychosocial problems in 3 patients.

Special Problems:

Patient No. 1:

A 12-year-old boy who was walking well with his orthoses fell and
sustained a fracture of the distal femur.   He was treated with a long
leg cast with the knee in extension and could walk again shortly after
the injury.   Thus, his fracture did not appear to shorten the period he
was able to walk.

Patient No. 2:

One patient ceased walking although he did not seem to have
deteriorated significantly.   However, his family felt that it was too
much of a burden to help the patient apply the braces every day, as they
had other children to look after.   With the abandonment of the
orthoses, the patient could not walk safely.   At home, he could walk by
holding onto furniture.   It was felt that he could have continued
walking if his braces were applied on a daily basis thus, clearly the
ability of the family to co-operate is very important.

Spinal fusion

The average age at which spinal fusion was carried out in our patients
was 14 years 3 months.   Between 10 and 17 segments were fused in a
one-stage procedure.   Initially, Harrington rod instrumentation with
spinal fusion using iliac crest bone was carried out.   Twenty-five
patients had this procedure and fused without any significant problem.
The patients were mobilised shortly after surgery, but required a body
jacket (TLSO) for approximately 6 months.   When the Luque technique

became available, we successfully used it for the next 15 patients, who
could be mobilized within 3 days following surgery without external
support.   Operative  blood  loss  was  considerable  and  required
replacement.   There were no deaths and the complications were  minimal.
Tracheostomies  were  carried  out when the vital capacity was less than
30% or when the ability to cough and raise tracheo-bronchial  secretions
was lost.   Two year follow-up after surgery did not reveal any pain, or
pseudarthrosis in the spine.   These  patients  did  not  lose  function
post-operatively  and  in  many  instances regained upright use of their
hands for table-top activities, and self-care improved.


## DISCUSSION


### Lower extremity contractures:
When DMD children become wheelchair dependent, flexion  contractures  at
the  hips  and  at the knees increase.   As most of their activities are
carried out in a wheelchair, these contractures are acceptable  and  hip
and  knee  releases  are  not  indicated.   However, persistent fixed
equinovarus contractures of the ankles and feet can lead to:
  (i)   Pain.
  (ii)  The development of pressure sores on the lateral side of the
        foot and in places where the foot is in contact with the
        wheelchair.
  (iii) The inability to wear shoes.
  When these secondary problems occur, ankle and foot releases  may  be
required  on feet that are no longer "functional" (Williams et al. 1984,
Hsu and Jackson 1985).


### Osteoporosis and fractures:
Gross  demineralization  occurs  in  patients  with  Duchenne  muscular
dystrophy,  and  is  more  marked with inactivity.   Fractures can occur
with minimal force.   Although the pain  usually  does  not  last  long,
these  fractures  need  to  be treated by additional immobilization (Hsu
1979).


### Spinal Deformity:
Duchenne muscular dystrophy patients who stand and walk generally do not

develop a fixed spinal curve. Spinal orthoses are discouraged in ambulatory patients. Prolonged standing and walking seems to delay the development of a fixed curvature. Despite support of the spine with a back support system incorporated in a wheelchair, spinal collapse is seen with advancing age. This is more marked in the younger child. Progressive spinal collapse usually is the indication for spinal bracing, spinal fusion or a combination of both (Lehman et al. 1986).

Ventilation:

Because of recent developments promoting survival from respiratory failure, the overall management of the older child with DMD needed to be reviewed. In the past, tracheal intubation and tracheostomy has only been carried out in unusual circumstances. This allowed for continued ventilation of the affected children whose muscles were so weak that they could not properly ventilate themselves and occasionally was used so that a major operation could be accomplished. These developments led to requests from the patient and/or his family for a permanent tracheostomy prior to the need for emergency measures. With these methods, the life-span of the DMD child has doubled (Gilgoff 1986). Thus secondary problems which were tolerable with a very much abbreviated life-span could no longer be accepted by the patient or his family. Prolonged ambulation lessens the severity of the secondary complications and the degree of demineralization (Hsu 1979). This coupled with surgical intervention in the ankles and feet and/or spine as required has become desirable and should be a part of the overall management regimen of the muscular dystrophy child.

## SUMMARY

(1) A programme to prolong ambulation and to delay permanent wheelchair sitting was carried out in 25 children with follow-up from 8 to 14 years.

(2) Prolongation of standing and walking was possible with this group of patients. The average prolongation of walking was 3·3 years.

(3) Secondary problems in a patient with Duchenne muscular dystrophy lead to pain, further loss of function, spinal deformity and pathological fractures. Prevention is highly desirable.

(4)    Spinal fusion is indicated for progressive spinal collapse.

REFERENCES

Carlson, J. M. and Winter, R. (1978). The 'Gillette' sitting support orthosis. Orthotics and Prosthetics, 32:  35-45.


Endo, H. (1969).  A study of bracing for patients with muscular dystrophy. Journal of West Pacific Orthopaedic Association, 6:  97-107.


Falewski de Leon, G. (1977). Maintenance of mobility. Israel Journal of Medical Science, 13:  177-182.


Galasko, C. S. B. (1986). The Duchenne muscular dystrophy child - care of the ambulatory patient. Muscle and Nerve, 9 (Supplement):  85.


Gardner-Medwin, D. (1979). Controversies about Duchenne muscular dystrophy. (2) Bracing for ambulation. Developmental Medicine and Child Neurology, 21:  659-662.


Gibson, D. A. Albisser, A. M. and Koreska, J. (1975). Role of the wheelchair in the management of the muscular dystrophy patient. Canadian Medical Association Journal, 113:  964-966.


Gilgoff, I. S. (1986). The respirator-dependent, neuromuscular patient. Muscle and Nerve, 9 (Supplement):  86.


Hsu, J. D. (1976). Management of foot deformity in Duchenne's pseudohypertrophic muscular dystrophy. Orthopaedic Clinics of North America, 7:  979-984.


Hsu, J. D. (1979). Extremity fractures in children with neuromuscular disease. John Hopkins Medical Journal, 145:  89-93.


Hsu, J. D. (1983). The natural history of spine curvature progression in the non-ambulatory Duchenne muscular dystrophy patient. Spine, 8: 771-775.

Hsu, J. D. (1986). The mid-80's - advances in technology for the care of the neuromuscular patient. Muscle and Nerve, 9 (Supplement): 85.

Hsu, J. D. and Jackson, R. (1985). Treatment of symptomatic foot and ankle deformities in the non-ambulatory neuromuscular patient. Foot and Ankle, 5: 238-244.

Lehman, M., Hsu, A. M. and Hsu, J. D. (1986). Spinal curvature, hand dominance and prolonged upper-extremity use of wheelchair-dependent DMD patients. Developmental Medicine and Child Neurology, 28: 628-632.

Pirot, J. (1972). Clinical studies in progressive muscular dystrophy. Polish Medical Journal, 11: 1004-1012.

Rideau, Y. Glorion, B. , Delaubier, A., Tarlé, O. and Bach, J. (1984). The treatment of scoliosis in Duchenne muscular dystrophy. Muscle and Nerve, 7: 281-286.

Roy, L. and Gibson, D. A. (1970). Pseudohypertrophic muscular dystrophy and its surgical management: Review of 30 patients. Canadian Journal of Surgery, 13: 13-21.

Sakai, D. N., Hsu, J. D., Bonnett, C. A. and Brown, J. C. (1977). Stabilization of the collapsing spine in Duchenne muscular dystrophy. Clinical Orthopaedics and Related Research, 128: 256-260.

Seeger, B. R., Caudrey, D. J. and Little, J. D. (1985). Progression of equinus deformity in Duchenne muscular dystrophy. Archives of Physical Medical Rehabilitation, 66: 286-288.

Shapiro, F. and Bresnan, M. J. (1982). Current concepts review - orthopaedic management of childhood neuromuscular disease. Part III: Diseases of muscle. Journal of Bone and Joint Surgery, 64-A: 1102-1107.

Siegel, I. M. (1972). Equinocavovarus in muscular dystrophy. Its treatment by percutaneous tarsal medullostomy and soft tissue release. Archives of Surgery, 104: 644-646.

Siegel, I. M. (1982). Spinal stabilization in Duchenne muscular dystrophy: Rationale and method. Muscle and Nerve, 5: 417-418.

Spencer, G. E. Jr. (1973). Orthopaedic considerations in the management of muscular dystrophy. Current Practices of Orthopaedic Surgery, 5: 279-293.

Sutherland, D. H., Olshen, R., Cooper, L., Wyatt, M., Leach, J., Mubarak, S. and Schultz, P. (1981). The patho-mechanics of gait in Duchenne muscular dystrophy. Developmental Medicine and Child Neurology, 23: 3-22.

Swank, S. M., Brown, J. C. and Perry, R. E. (1982). Spinal fusion in Duchenne muscular dystrophy. Spine, 7: 484-491.

Williams, E. A., Read, L., Ellis, A., Morris, P. and Galasko, C. S. B. (1984). The management of equinus deformity in Duchenne muscular dystrophy. Journal of Bone and Joint Surgery, 66-B: 546-550.

Young, A., Johnson, D., O'Gorman, E., MacMillan, T. and Chase, A. P. (1984). A new spinal brace for use in Duchenne muscular dystrophy. Developmental Medicine and Child Neurology, 26: 808-813.

## 25.SPINAL CORD MONITORING DURING SURGERY FOR SCOLIOSIS

M. Arafa
P. Morris
C. S. B. Galasko

### INTRODUCTION

The surgical correction of spinal deformities with a distraction force, as in Harrington or Luque instrumentation, carries a small but significant risk of neurological complications due to iatrogenic injuries to the spinal cord. A survey conducted by the Scoliosis Research Society found 87 patients with acute neurological complications resulting from the treatment of scoliosis: an overall incidence of 0·72% (MacEwen et al. 1975).

In order to reduce the incidence of such problems, several methods of evaluating spinal cord function have been introduced. The "wake up" test and somatosensory evoked potentials (SEP) recordings are both used in the intra-operative assessment of spinal cord function during spinal surgery.

Vauzelle and associates (1973), and Hall and co-workers (1978) reported the use of the "wake up" test in 124 and 166 patients respectively. No untoward complications were encountered in either series. The test relies on the patient's understanding and co-operation and is contraindicated in patients with psychological problems, mental retardation, or who are very young. There are possible hazards in arousing an intubated patient from anaesthesia, with the patient lying prone on a frame including accidental extubation, pulmonary aeroembolism due to aspiration of air into the open vessels in the wound, and dislodgement of the rod during a violent movement.

The rationale for monitoring sensory evoked responses during spinal surgery is to detect and hopefully reverse untoward effects resulting from ischaemia, distortion or possible disruption of critical neural pathways.

There are two basic techniques for applying the stimulus. Direct stimulation of the spinal cord by means of a small, bipolar, epidural electrode has been favoured by some groups (Tsuyama et al. 1978). They presume that the high amplitude waveforms reflect the activity of both the sensory and motor fibres. However, the direct stimulation of the spinal cord could result in heating effects on cord tissues or biochemical changes.

Stimulation of peripheral mixed nerves by large electrodes attached to the skin is an alternative technique (Jones et al. 1982, 1983). It is safe, allows lateralised testing, and has been shown to produce low amplitude but otherwise satisfactory recordings.

The sensory signals evoked by peripheral nerve stimulation can be recorded by means of electrodes glued to the scalp over the somatosensory cortex (Dawson 1947), inserted into the vertebral bone (Nordwall et al. 1979), or into the epidural space (Jones et al. 1982).

The cortical SEP clearly would be the method of choice since it could be used pre-, intra-, and post-operatively if required. A rather slow stimulation rate must be used, thus prolonging the time needed to acquire a set of readings, but the primary difficulty with this technique is the depressive effect of anaesthetic agents on the cortical SEP (Jones et al. 1982, Bradshaw et al. 1984).

Using electrodes designed for insertion into vertebral bone, it has been shown that spinal cord potentials can be recorded from the spinous process. However, compared with other techniques, the amplitude is reduced by 50% and the technique is less reliable at high thoracic and cervical regions (Bradshaw et al. 1984).

The available evidence tends to favour epidural techniques as providing the most reliable recording method (Jones et al. 1982, Bradshaw et al. 1984).


## PATIENTS AND METHODS

This report describes our experience with epidural spinal SEP in 29 patients who underwent spinal surgery for scoliosis at the Royal Manchester Children's Hospital, between December 1984 and September 1986. There were 18 males and 11 females. The average age was 13 years (range 8-19 years). The scoliosis was idiopathic in 12 patients, congenital in 2 patients and neuromuscular in 15 patients.    Harrington instrumentation was used in 13 patients and the Luque system was used in 16 patients.    The average pre-operative curve was 56° (range   14-103°). The average post-operative curve was 35° (range 7-78°).    All patients had a full pre-operative cardiac and respiratory assessment.

The anaesthetic regimen was as follows:   Lorazepam (2·5 mg) and Droperidol (5·0 mg) were used as a premedication;   Thiopentone (5 mg/Kgm bodyweight) and Fentanyl (2 mg/Kgm bodyweight) were used for  induction. A non depolarising neuroblocking agent was used as a muscle relaxant. The anaesthetic was maintained with 70% Nitrous Oxide,   30%   Oxygen and volatile Halothane or Isofleuran.

Evoked potentials were recorded in the operating room by Medelec Monitor 91.   The stimulus electrodes were placed at the popliteal fossa, overlying the right and left posterior tibial nerves.   An earthing electrode was secured to one thigh.   The stimulus was provided by a square-wave electrical impulse of duration 0·2 milliseconds and intensity between 25 and 150 volts (usually 100  volts),   sufficient to produce a direct motor response in the foot.   This was delivered at a rate of 2, 10, or 20 per second, according to the nature of the response to be recorded.

The epidural electrode consisted of a one meter braided stainless steel electrode coated with polytetrafluoroethylene (PTFE)   and   capped with pure platinum to produce a smooth tip of 1·3 millimetre diameter and 17 square millimetre surface area.   The reference electrode had  a similar lead construction with a stainless steel needle.

After exposure of the vertebrae, the epidural electrode was introduced above the upper level of instrumentation into   the   epidural space and advanced 1-3 cms cephalad.   The reference electrode was inserted into muscle alongside the epidural recording site.

Comparison of current response of the cord to the previously recorded "control" trace was achieved by obtaining a stable response from the patient prior to any cord manipulation.

The recording was usually obtained at the space between the second and third dorsal vertebrae.   At this level the waveform usually consisted of three components.   The latencies of the three negative potentials were approximately 15, 17, and 19 milliseconds (Figure 1). The earliest potential (N15) probably represented activity in the dorsal spinocerebellar tracts.   The later potentials may have been due to activity in the posterior columns.

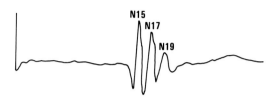

FIG. 1.  Normal recording (see text).

Changes in the epidural response, indicating cord dysfunction usually take the form of a complete ablation of the response.  Occasionally, changes in latency or amplitude may indicate spinal cord distress.

RESULTS

No responses could be recorded from one patient with spina bifida, one patient with Friedreich's ataxia and one patient with peripheral neuropathy (Figure 2).

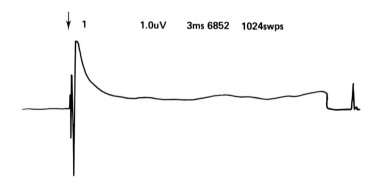

FIG. 2.  Patient with peripheral neuropathy.  No epidural response was recorded to posterior tibial nerve stimulation.

In one patient there was bilateral flattening of the waveform during the final stage of Luque instrumentation.  However, on loosening the responsible sublaminar wires a normal trace returned.  There was

no residual post-operative neurological deficit (Figure 3). The
responses remained normal throughout the procedure in the other 25
patients.

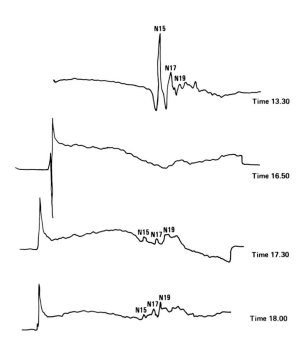

FIG. 3. Patient with cerebral palsy. The waveform was lost during the
final stage of Luque instrumentation, but returned on loosening the
responsible sublaminar wires.


## DISCUSSION

Our results confirm that epidural spinal SEP is sensitive to minor
spinal cord impairment, and that these changes may be reversed when the
cause is quickly remedied. The monitoring system interfered minimally
with the anaesthetic or surgical procedure and should be used as a
routine. However, the technique may not be reliable in some patients
with neuromuscular scoliosis, such as spina bifida, Friedreich's ataxia
and the neuropathies.

REFERENCES

Bradshaw, K., Webb, J. K. and Fraser, A. M. (1984). Clinical evaluation of spinal cord monitoring in scoliosis surgery. Spine, 9: 636-643.

Dawson, G. D. (1947). Cerebral responses to electrical stimulation of peripheral nerve in man. Journal of Neurology, Neurosurgery and Psychiatry, 10: 134-140.

Hall, J. E., Levine, C. R. and Sudhir, K. G. (1978). Intraoperative awakening to monitor spinal cord function during Harrington instrumentation and spine fusion. Journal of Bone and Joint Surgery, 60-A: 533-536.

Jones, S. J., Edgar, M. A. and Ransford, A. D. (1982). Sensory nerve conduction in the human spinal cord: epidural recordings made during scoliosis surgery. Journal of Neurology, Neurosurgery and Psychiatry, 45: 446-451.

Jones, S. J., Edgar, M. A., Ransford, A. D. and Thomas, N. P. (1983). A system for the electrophysiological monitoring of the spinal cord during operations for scoliosis. Journal of Bone and Joint Surgery, 65-B: 134-139.

MacEwen, G. D., Bunnell, W. P. and Sriram, K. (1975). Acute neurological complications in the treatment of scoliosis: A report of the Scoliosis Research Society. Journal of Bone and Joint Surgery, 57-A: 404-408.

Nordwall, A., Axelgaard, J., Harada, Y., Valencia, P., McNeal, D. R. and Brown, J. C. (1979). Spinal cord monitoring using evoked potentials recorded from feline vertebral bone. Spine, 4: 486-494.

Tsuyama, N., Tsuzuki, N., Kurokawa, T. and Imai, T. (1978). Clinical application of spinal cord action potential measurement. International Orthopaedics, 2: 39-46.

Vauzelle, C., Stagnara, P. and Jouvinroux, P. (1973). Functional
monitoring of spinal cord activity during spinal surgery. Clinical
Orthopaedics and Related Research, 93: 173-178.

## 26. MODERN TRENDS IN THE TRANSFER OF ORTHOPAEDIC PATIENTS BY AIR

A. Hughes
N. Toff

Over the last 10-15 years there has been a rapid increase in the use of civil aircraft for medical purposes in the United Kingdom. This has been fuelled by the huge rise in the number of holidaymakers travelling abroad and by their expectation of a swift repatriation by "air ambulance" should any medical misfortune befall them. The aim of this paper is to place this work in context, to present an estimate of the numbers involved and briefly to discuss some of the problems associated with the transfer by air of patients with musculo-skeletal trauma. The history of evacuation of patients by air follows the time honoured sequence of invention by genius, development by warmongers and finally, adoption by peace abiding civilians. The genius of the Montgolfiers in 1783 led to the use of balloons in the European wars for observing enemy troops and, in 1890, to what is often cited as the first use of an air ambulance, when 150 wounded French soldiers were evacuated by balloon during the seige of Paris. The invention of the Wright brothers appeared in 1903 when Sir Harry Platt was 17 years old, and, even before the Great War, was being modified for the carriage of patients. During the final months of that war some use was made of the aeroplane for the evacuation of wounded soldiers but it was not to come into its own as an ambulance until the next major conflict.

The rotary wing technology of the late 1930's was not sufficiently developed to produce much impact in World War II, but in Korea and then in Vietnam, helicopters proved indispensable in taking medical care to the front line and in "scoop and fly" missions to remove the severely injured to the MASH units.

In peacetime, civilian air transfer of trauma patients is valuable in two settings (Figure 1).

Firstly, the primary evacuation of patients from the scene of injury to the site of definitive medical care. There is no doubt that the survival of the most seriously injured is increased by rapid removal, although there continues to be debate as to whether it is the early intervention by the flown-in medical team at the scene of the accident or the earlier hospitalization which has led to a reduction in patient mortality.

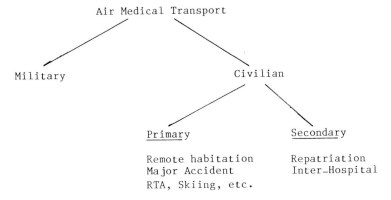

FIG. 1.    Role of civilian air transfer.

On the continent, particularly in Switzerland, Germany and France, there are well developed and integrated helicopter ambulance services which compliment the usual ground services. In the U.K., the fixed wing aircraft which operate to the islands and remote areas of Scotland act, when necessary, as air ambulances, funded by the N.H.S. However, apart from a small experimental scheme in Devon and Cornwall, the only helicopter service is that provided by the R.A.F. and Royal Navy Search and Rescue Units. Whether a national civilian helicopter service, such as exists on the continent, could be justified or implemented in this country remains to be seen. The high level of commitment, both financial and political, makes this seem unlikely at present.

The second area of value of air transfer, and that which mainly concerns this paper, is the secondary transfer of patients, most importantly in terms of numbers, from abroad, but also within the U.K.

The development of the civil jet airliner and the advent of cheap air travel has seen an explosive growth in tourism and business travel. Approximately 800 million passengers travel by air each year and the volume has been increasing steadily by 3-5% per year during the 1980's.

Heathrow alone coped with 30 million passengers and it has been estimated that 22 million British citizens spent at least one day abroad last year (Table 1).

### Table 1:  Scale of Foreign Travel

22 Million Britons travelled abroad in 1985

(approximately 16 Million tourists)

3 - 5% increase per annum

1% claimed on insurance policies

0·1% required medical assistance

The majority of tourists are covered by some form of medical insurance and it is the insurers who are funding the bulk of the medical air transfers, the execution of which is normally delegated to a medical assistance or air ambulance company.

The insurers, assistance companies and aircraft operators have good commercial reasons for keeping the detailed statistics relating to their operations a closely guarded secret and since no official agency keeps figures of air ambulance transfers, it is difficult to know the numbers of trauma patients involved.

We have attempted to produce some "ball park" figures for the totals by combining the results of our own surveys with informed estimates of the market volume (Table 2).

### Table 2:  Estimated Volume of Air Transfers to the U.K. per annum

| | | | |
|---|---|---|---|
| Total | – | 6500 | – 7000 |
| Dead | – | 350 | – 400 |
| Medical | – | 2400 | – 2800 |
| Surgical | – | 1000 | – 1200 |
| Psychiatric | – | | 300 |
| Obst./Gynae. | – | | 300 |
| Trauma | – | 1800 | – 2000 |

Of those who require or are granted an air transfer, the majority travel on a normal scheduled or charter flight, either in a seat or on a stretcher, accompanied or alone. Whether travelling in this way or aboard an air ambulance aircraft there are new influences on the patient and his injury which are particular to the environment of the aircraft cabin and which are absent on the ground, and in a hospital bed.

It is common knowledge that modern jet aircraft have pressurized cabins to protect the occupants from hypoxia and the decompression effects which otherwise would occur in the thin air at altitude. What is less often realized is that the cabin is not pressurized to sea level but to the equivalent of 6-8,000 feet in airline aircraft and 8-10,000 feet in the type of aircraft typically used for air ambulance flights. This enables a saving in weight, fuel, and, therefore, cost and is acceptable since there are no adverse physiological or psychological effects on the healthy human.

However, the injured patient may be affected in one of several ways. The reduction in inspired $PO_2$ will result in a reduced arterial $PO_2$. There may be serious consequences where there is already cardiovascular or respiratory impairment or if trauma has compromised tissue blood supply. Therefore, patients with soft tissue injuries, particularly in the region of highly "dependent" tissues such as those of the central nervous system, will require supplementary inspired oxygen.

The variation in cabin pressure itself may affect tissue swelling and it is a golden rule that cylinder plaster casts less than 48 hours old are split, or preferably bivalved, before flight and the limb circulation is carefully watched. Any gas trapped in a closed space will attempt to expand (up to 50% at 10,000 foot altitude) and this includes air trapped beneath plasters, in penetrating wounds, in facial sinuses, a pneumothorax or an ileus. Also affected are any air or vacuum splints, catheter balloons, etc.

A major risk to the trauma patient may be that of the movement involved in transfer by air. This includes the transfer on the ground, loading and unloading from the aircraft, as well as accelerations occurring during the flight. Careful attention to splintage, patient security and comfort are all important and, where applicable, internal fixation of fractures is preferred before flight. The usefulness of the vacuum mattress (and occasionally the MAS suit) in this context, often outweighs the disadvantages mentioned above but the use of traction splints involving weights is ineffective and dangerous.

Other factors in the aircraft environment are shown in Table 3.

Table 3:   Influences on Patient and Medical Equipment in Flight

Loading and Unloading

Reduced Cabin Pressure   - oxygenation
                          gas expansion

Environmental Stresses   - humidity
                          temperature
                          noise
                          vibration

Accelerations

Confined Space

Emotional Upheaval

Flight Emergencies

How  is the trauma patient transferred in practice?   Patients can be
divided simply into those who can sit in a seat - either walking  aboard
or assisted using a wheelchair - and those requiring a stretcher.

The  former  group  includes  those  with upper and distal lower limb
injuries.   Apart from the points  mentioned  above  and  provided  that
there  are  no  additional complicating factors, there is little to note
apart from emphasizing again the care that must be  taken  with  plaster
casts.    The  latter  group  includes  patients  with spinal fractures,
backache (including sciatic pain where pressure changes  are  likely  to
lead  to  further  oedema  around  the  nerve  root), pelvic and femoral
fractures.

There  is  no  place  for  a rapid but poorly planned transfer of any
patient and especially of patients with spinal injuries, who  have  been
the  subject  of mismanagement and the source of numerous horror stories
in the not-too-distant past.   If this is to be the case, such  patients
are safer left in their hospital bed no matter where it may be.   If the
facilities are available, the skeleton should be stabilized  by  correct
internal  fixation,  particularly  if  there  is a neurological deficit.
This  might  even  involve  "flying-in"  an  orthopaedic  surgeon  from
elsewhere.   The  second  best  option  is  to  stabilize  by  external
fixation.   There are stretchers which have been individually converted
so that  traction  may be applied to the cervical spine using  a  spring

balance but they are not in general use at present and so the use of tongs is precluded. Problems posed by such devices include the need to maintain adequate counter-traction during accelerations, the requirement that the patient should remain in traction during all phases of the transfer and the space required to accommodate the additional length aboard the aircraft. The Stryker turning frame would be one solution but aircraft large enough to accommodate this safely are also very expensive. The simplest safe method, therefore, is to use a halo jacket. It must be ensured that this is of the type where the jacket can be released if necessary to deal with respiratory or cardiac problems (Table 4).

### Table 4: Spinal Injuries

(A)     Plan the flight

(B)     Stabilise the skeleton        Internal fixation

                                      Stryker Frame + Traction

                                      Halo Jacket

                                      External Splint

                                      Vacuum Mattress

                                      Scoop Stretcher

(C)     Total body nursing

(D)     IVI and $O_2$

Patients with pelvic fractures must be fully resuscitated prior to flight. The hazard of delayed shock from concealed haemorrhage is a major risk in the early post injury period. It can also be one of the most awkward problems to deal with during flight due to the limited quantity of fluid, both colloid and crystalloid, which is available. Blood is not normally carried on board. The pelvis should be stabilized, even if already internally fixed, using a vacuum mattress or MAS suit, and an intravenous infusion should be in place (Table 5).

Femoral fracture is a common diagnosis among air ambulance patients and all ages are involved. Once again, the blood volume loss should be critically assessed and, if necessary, corrected prior to the flight. If not already fixed, limb traction can be easily and comfortably applied using a device such as the Donway traction splint which has all the ideal characteristics for use in the aircraft (Table 6).

### Table 5:  Pelvic Injuries

(A)    Plan the flight

(B)    Stabilise the skeleton        →    Internal fixation

External fixation

G suit

Vacuum mattress

Scoop stretcher

(C)    IVI and $O_2$

### Table 6:   Femoral Fractures (including Acetabular)

(A)    Plan the flight

(B)    Stabilise the skeleton        →    Internal fixation

Donway splint

G suit

Vacuum mattress

Scoop stretcher

(C)    IVI and $O_2$

In each instance, a careful assessment of the patient's injuries  and a good working knowledge of the effects of flight on the patient and the medical equipment is vital for the safety and comfort of the patient and for the peace of mind of the medical attendant.

It  has been predicted that industry will be in space during the next decade and tourists within a generation.   Plans for medical  evacuation from space already exist.

## 27. ROAD TRAUMA IN AUSTRALIA

### F. B. Webb

### INTRODUCTION

Whilst there is a little controversy regarding the date and who invented the petrol driven motor car, there is no argument that Daimler and Benz built the world's first four-wheeled petrol engine driven cars independently, although quite close to one another in 1886 and that 1986 is the centenary of the motor car. In 1888 Karl Benz retailed his 1·5 H.P. car, which marked the beginning of the motor industry when the American Orthopaedic Association was just one year old and Sir Harry Platt two years of age. The motor vehicle has dramatically changed our way of life in the western world during the past 100 years. We have become part-time crustaceans, often with a marked change in personality when we retreat into our shells – the mouse in the office, and the lion on the road. We work, go to work, play, compete, use as status symbols, court, sometimes are conceived, born or die in a motor vehicle, and for most of us our last journey on this earth will be in a motorised hearse. Our houses, cities, and highways are designed around the motor vehicle.

Road trauma has inexorably changed the face of orthopaedic surgery, and the change has escalated dramatically over the last 40 years since the end of World War II. Tuberculosis and poliomyelitis have virtually disappeared in the western world and those on whom Sir Harry did so much of his work have been replaced by the victims of road trauma. Although this paper is confined to road trauma in Australia, the epidemiological pattern is the same in Britain, Europe and the U.S.A. It is an endemic disease of major proportions, is the single largest cause of death and disability below the age of 40 years, and in terms of loss of life, the road toll ranks ahead of all other diseases. It is a community health

problem of enormous magnitude which affects each and every one of us.
It is a toll paid in blood and suffering.   It is no respecter of  race,
age, religion, creed or politics (Tables 1 and 2).

Table 1

1984 ROAD DEATHS
PER 100,000 POPULATION

| | |
|---|---|
| YUGOSLAVIA | 23·4 |
| AUSTRIA | 23·1 |
| BELGIUM | 21·2 |
| NEW ZEALAND | 20·2 |
| FRANCE | 19·7 |
| U.S.A. | 18·7 |
| AUSTRALIA | 18·2 |
| WEST GERMANY | 16·7 |
| CANADA | 15·5 |
| UNITED KINGDOM | 10·1 |
| SWEDEN | 9·6 |
| JAPAN | 7·7 |

Table 2

1983 ROAD DEATHS

PER 100 X $10^6$ VEHICLE Kms TRAVELLED

| | |
|---|---|
| NEW ZEALAND | 3·7 |
| GERMANY | 3·4 |
| AUSTRALIA | 2·4 |
| JAPAN | 2·4 |
| CANADA | 2·3 |
| UNITED KINGDOM | 2·1 |
| SWEDEN | 1·8 |
| U.S.A. | 1·6 |

Approximately 70% of those severely injured on the road are cared for by Orthopaedic Surgeons and although Orthopaedic Surgeons in training are taught how to manage the injured victim, little or nothing is taught about the epidemiology of the disease.

Table 3

ROAD DEATHS IN AUSTRALIA

|  | 1984 | 1985 | CHANGE | % CHANGE |
|---|---|---|---|---|
| AUSTRALIA | 2,824 | 2,927 | ↑103 | +3·6% |
| WESTERN AUSTRALIA | 221 | 243 | ↑ 21 | + 10% |
| NEW SOUTH WALES | 1,037 | 1,066 | ↑ 29 | +2·8% |
| VICTORIA | 657 | 671 | ↑ 14 | +2·1% |
| QUEENSLAND | 505 | 502 | ↓ 3 | − 1% |
| SOUTH AUSTRALIA | 232 | 268 | ↑ 36 | +15·5% |
| TASMANIA | 84 | 77 | ↓ 7 | −8·3% |
| NORTHERN TERRITORIES | 50 | 67 | ↑ 17 | + 34% |
| AUSTRALIAN CAPITAL TERRITORY | 38 | 33 | ↓ 5 | −13·2% |

Table 4

ROAD DEATHS IN AUSTRALIA

|  | JANUARY–JUNE '85 | JANUARY–JUNE '86 |
|---|---|---|
| AUSTRALIA | 1,393 | 1,489 |
| WESTERN AUSTRALIA | 116 | 133 |
| NEW SOUTH WALES | 483 | 533 |
| VICTORIA | 336 | 351 |
| QUEENSLAND | 253 | 255 |
| SOUTH AUSTRALIA | 119 | 122 |
| TASMANIA | 41 | 39 |
| NORTHERN TERRITORIES | 28 | 38 |
| AUSTRALIAN CAPITAL TERRITORY | 17 | 18 |

Table 5

ROAD TRAUMA IN U.K.

|  | TOTAL CASUALTIES | KILLED | SERIOUSLY INJURED | SLIGHTLY INJURED |
|---|---|---|---|---|
| 1984 | 324,314 | 5,599 | 73,059 | 245,656 |
| 1985 | 317,524 | 5,165 | 70,980 | 241,379 |

Table 6

ROAD TRAUMA IN U.K.

|  | TOTAL CASUALTIES | KILLED | SERIOUSLY INJURED | SLIGHTLY INJURED |
|---|---|---|---|---|
| 1985 1st QUARTER | 65,510 | 1,071 | 14,489 | 49,950 |
| 1986 1st QUARTER | 69,012 | 1,122 | 14,888 | 53,002 |

INCIDENCE

The population of Australia is about 15 million, of whom 100,000 are injured and 2,500–3,000 killed per year on the roads.

Every 18 minutes an Australian is seriously injured, every 3 hours someone is killed and approximately 80 are hospitalized each day as a result of a road traffic accident. Motor cycle riders have a 6 times greater risk of death or injury.

Australia has been engaged in four wars since 1939:- the Second World War, Korea, the Malaysian Emergency and Vietnam. For every Australian killed in war, 1·6 have died on Australian roads; and for every Australian wounded, 5·8 have been injured on the roads during the same period by their own countrymen. The road deaths for 1984 were 2,824 and for 1985, 2,917 - a rise of 103 or 3·6% with a substantial rise of 15·5% in South Australia and a massive 34% increase in the Northern Territory which has the highest per capita beer consumption in the country (Table 3). The road deaths for the six months January to June increased from 1,393 in 1985 to 1,489 in 1986 (Table 4). Seventy per cent of the deaths were due to neuro-trauma, but the major concern is the ever-increasing number of the mentally and physically crippled who are not included in the statistics. The total cost to the Australian community is in excess of

3 billion dollars annually and the average cost to the community is in excess of $60,000 per crash. The average cost of loss of production with each road death of 15-24 year olds is $434,000.

The figures for the U.K. are similar (Tables 5 and 6). Although there was a decrease from 1984 to 1985, the figures for the first quarter of 1986 showed an increase.


## PREVENTION

The problems and the solutions are multi-factorial, but there are two main factors - Youth and Alcohol. At a blood alcohol concentration of ·02%, alcohol adversely affected judgement ability, an ability which is essential for safe driving (Drew et al. 1958). Action is required to reduce the road toll, including better education and more effective legislation. The Royal Australasian College of Surgeons have been active in the fight against road trauma since 1970. There is no doubt that Victoria has led Australia in the matter of effective legislation, but New South Wales is catching up. The concept that accidents always happen to other people must be dispelled. In Australia, there is a one in four chance that a member of a typical four unit family will be killed or injured, not just involved, in a traffic accident during the next 10 years. Albert Sabin did more for orthopaedics in developing a poliomyelitis vaccine than any Orthopaedic Surgeon. Prevention is so much better than cure and Orthopaedic Surgeons must play an active role to help reduce the road toll.


## REFERENCES

Drew, G. C., Colquhoun, W. P. and Long, H. A. (1958). Effect of small doses of alcohol on a skill resembling driving. British Medical Journal, 2: 993-999.

Cohen, J., Dearnaley, E. J. and Hansel, C. E. M. (1958). The risk taken in driving under the influence of alcohol. British Medical Journal, 1: 1438-1442.

# 28

ADVANCES  IN  DIAGNOSIS  AND TREATMENT OF CLOSED TRACTION LESIONS OF THE
BRACHIAL PLEXUS

R. Birch

## INTRODUCTION

Platt (1921) recorded important observations  from  the  study  of  such
techniques  of  nerve  repair  as grafting and tubulisation, and, later,
discussed the question of obstetrical paralysis (Platt 1973).

   This paper summarises experience with 1,000 patients with lesions  of
the brachial plexus seen since 1977 (Tables 1 and 2) and concentrates on
problems of diagnosis and treatment of patients  suffering  from  closed
traction lesion of the brachial plexus.   There are a significant number
of patients suffering from iatrogenic lesions of  the  brachial  plexus;
from  errors  at  operation  in  the  posterior  triangle  of  the neck,
following irradiation of  the  axilla  and  neck  in  the  treatment  of
malignant neoplastic disease, and a steady increase in birth palsies.

## PROBLEMS OF DIAGNOSIS IN CLOSED TRACTION LESION OF THE BRACHIAL PLEXUS

The  cult of the motorcycle has led to an epidemic of crippling injuries
of the upper  limb  in  young  people.   In  most  cases  the  head  is
distracted  from  the  upper limb and the brachial plexus often fails at
its weakest point;  the attachment of the spinal nerves  to  the  spinal
cord.   The extent of involvement of the brachial plexus is evident from
simple clinical examination;  determination of the level of  lesion  may
prove  more  difficult.   Abrasions  on  the  chin,  the  neck, and the
shoulder demonstrate a violent distraction of the upper  limb  from  the
head  and  neck.   Deep  bruising in the posterior triangle of the neck
indicates injury to the great vessels but  also  severe  injury  to  the
paravertebral muscles.   Sensory  loss extending above the clavicle is a

## Table 1

Findings and procedures in 576 patients undergoing operation for lesions of the supraclavicular brachial plexus.

|    |                                                                                                              | Number of patients |
|----|--------------------------------------------------------------------------------------------------------------|:------------------:|
| 1. | Complete preganglionic lesion of brachial plexus                                                             | 78                 |
| 2. | Pre-ganglionic injury of one or more spinal roots, with sparing of the other roots                          | 97                 |
| 3. | Repair of supraclavicular lesion of the brachial plexus by standard nerve grafting, by nerve transfer or by direct suture | 105 |
| 4. | Repair by vascularised ulnar nerve graft                                                                     | 49                 |
| 5. | Reconstructive operations                                                                                    | 203                |
|    | (In many of these patients more than one operation was carried out; in one half previous exploration with or without repair had been performed) | |
| 6. | Irradiation neuritis                                                                                         | 18                 |
| 7. | Tumour                                                                                                       | 26                 |

## Table 2

Repairs of vessels and nerves in 94 patients with infraclavicular lesion

| | |
|---|:---:|
| Patients in whom neural repair carried out | 50 |
| Patients with repair of axillary vessels | 43 |
| Number of recognised ruptures of nerve trunks | 121 |
| Number of repairs of nerve trunks | 79 |

bad sign, indicating involvement of the upper cervical roots, and paralysis of the thoraco-scapular muscles including trapezius and serratus anterior is further evidence of this. A Claude Bernard-Horner syndrome, and pain felt in the anaesthetic hand suggests proximal injury to the eighth cervical and first thoracic roots. Plain radiographs of the cervical spine and of the chest are valuable. Avulsion of the transverse processes of the sixth and seventh cervical verebrae is almost always associated with avulsion of the spinal nerves at that

level.    Fracture  dislocation  of  the first rib is usually associated
with avulsion of the first thoracic root;  elevation of the  ipsilateral
diaphragm confirms injury to the phrenic nerve.

After  about  3  weeks  Wallerian degeneration will have occurred and
from this time the investigations developed by Bonney are of great value
(Bonney  1954,  Bonney  and  Gilliatt 1958), but there are difficulties.
There is much variation in the somatotomes of the  upper  limb  and  the
fifth  cervical nerve is difficult to sample;  it is not easy to observe
the Histamine response in hairy or pigmented skin;  and there  may  have
been a distal injury to a nerve trunk.

Myelography  is  valuable  but computerised tomographic scanning with
contrast enhancement is more accurate, particularly for the 5th and  6th
cervical  nerves  (Marshall  and  De  Silva, in  press).   We have very
limited experience with  magnetic  resonance  imaging but  this  seems
promising.   Demonstration of evoked cortical sensory potentials, before
and during operation gives further information (Jones et al. 1981).

Whilst all these investigations  contribute  to  accurate  diagnosis,
anatomic variations and distal nerve ruptures can be misleading.


## INDICATIONS FOR OPERATION AND TECHNIQUES OF REPAIR

Operation  is  indicated  to establish the diagnosis and to repair nerve
ruptures if these  are  suspected.   Vascular  injuries  demand  urgent
operation.   Early  exploration  in  patients with dense lesions of the
brachial plexus is valuable because the  dissection  is  usually  easier
before  oedema  and  fibrosis  mar  the field, and stimulation of distal
nerve stumps is helpful in detecting predominantly motor bundles and  to
exclude  concealed  distal  rupture  of nerve trunks.   The diagnosis is
established early and appropriate reconstructive operations are  planned
before  the  patient  becomes psychologically one handed (Narakas 1978).
The results of early repair of nerve ruptures by graft are substantially
better  than  in  patients  where there has been delay.   Where patients
present after a delay of some weeks the presence of a static Tinel  sign
with  radiation into the appropriate somatotome is a good indication for
exploration  in  the  anticipation  of  finding  a  reparable  lesion.
Electromyography  of the deltoid and of the biceps at about three months
in a patient with persisting paralysis of these muscles is useful.

The prepared field should include the whole of the upper limb and also the lower limbs to allow access to the sural nerve. The plexus is formally exposed by a transverse supraclavicular incision. Following section of the scalenus anterior the lower trunk and subclavian artery are exposed. Neuromuscular blocking agents are avoided during induction to allow the use of the nerve stimulator.

Modes of repair are dictated by the findings at operation. Although direct suture is possible if a nerve has been transected by a knife such direct suture is never possible in a traction lesion. Transfer of a ruptured root proximally to a distal stump is possible in early cases before retraction has occurred but in the great majority of patients repair is effected by standard interfascicular grafting using cutaneous nerve grafts. In patients where the prognosis for the ulnar nerve is demonstrated to be hopeless, a vascularised ulnar nerve graft is used and we now prefer the segment of the nerve in the arm based on the superior ulnar collateral vessels to the 'classical' ulnar nerve graft (Bonney at al. 1984), using the nerve in the forearm based on the ulnar vessels. Intercostal nerve transfer is of limited value; we reserve it for children and for adults where there has been recovery through the lower trunk, who have the potential for function in the hand and in whom there is no possible mode of restoring elbow flexion.

## The infraclavicular lesion

Infraclavicular lesions of the brachial plexus form 20% of our series. The cause is hyperextension of the shoulder and fracture of the scapula or humerus is usual. Nearly 50% of our patients have ruptured their axillary artery. The case for early exploration and primary repair is particularly strong in these patients, since delay leads to irredeemable marring of the limb from ischaemic fibrosis. Lesions vary from simple ruptures of isolated nerves, such as the musculocutaneous or axillary nerves, to wide ruptures of all of the trunk nerves of the limb. We believe that the proper treatment of these injuries includes stabilisation of the skeleton, restoration of circulation, adequate decompression and primary grafting of nerve ruptures.

## RESULTS

The prognosis for function of a limb following a severe lesion of the brachial plexus is bad. It is rare for a patient to use the limb in a normal manner. The outcome of repair of predominantly motor nerves such as axillary and musculocutaneous is generally good and restoration of some degree of control of the shoulder joint and of elbow flexion is usual. Significant return of function into the forearm and hand occurs only in the youngest patients. Delay in repair diminishes the final functional result. The use of the limb may be enhanced considerably by appropriate muscle or tendon transfers or, in selected cases, by arthrodesis of the glenohumeral joint. Such reconstructive operations are particularly indicated in partial lesions of the brachial plexus. Once the diagnosis has been established such operations should not be delayed.

Detailed discussion of modes of reconstruction is inappropriate in this paper, but we would emphasise that transfer of latissimus dorsi to the upper and outer aspect of the humerus is particularly valuable in children with birth injuries to the upper trunk if contracture at the shoulder joint has not occurred. Many of these children regain normal co-ordination and cadence of shoulder movement. In adults, however, muscle transfers to restore shoulder control are unpredictable and in well motivated adults with good hand function gleno-humeral fusion is a particularly beneficial operation.

Loss of elbow flexion is particularly disabling and although the Steindler operation is most frequently performed, transfer of pectoralis major or of latissimus dorsi has enhanced function in many. Transfer of triceps to biceps is useful when co-contraction between these two antagonists cannot be overcome. It should be remembered that latissimus dorsi is an ideal muscle to restore elbow extension. The most commonly performed operation for reconstruction is flexor to extensor tendon transfer. In the great majority of patients the lesion involves the fifth, sixth and seventh cervical nerves, and there is paralysis of pronator teres. Results from high median transfer, where brachioradialis or extensor carpi radialis longus are used to restore flexion of the digits remind us of the importance of sensory function in the hand. Indeed patients with irreparable lesions of the fifth and sixth cervical nerves appear to be more disabled than those with preganglionic injury of the eighth cervical and the first thoracic nerves. The last group have normal shoulder and elbow function with good sensation in the thumb, index and middle fingers. Tendon transfers within the hand are only indicated in patients with good proximal function and in whom sensation in the hand has been largely spared.

## REHABILITATION

The majority of our patients are manual workers and the dominant limb is usually afflicted. Treatment of these patients must be guided by the need to enable them to return to some useful social existence and this demands prompt diagnosis, early repair of nerve, or early muscle or tendon transfer where appropriate. Orthoses such as the flail arm splint are often valuable. Pain is a serious problem for patients with a lesion of the brachial plexus, and on occasion it is the overwhelming problem (Wynn Parry 1981). Treatment is difficult; the transcutaneous nerve stimulator is useful for many and is certainly preferable to addiction to alcohol or to opiates. For most patients, return to a useful occupation is the most important factor in adapting to pain. In a small minority ablation of the dorsal root entry zone may be considered but the hazards of these operations are considerable.

## REFERENCES

Bonney, G. (1954). Value of axon responses in determining site of lesion in traction injuries of the brachial plexus. Brain, 77: 588-609.

Bonney, G. and Gilliatt, R. W. (1958). Sensory nerve conduction after traction lesion of the brachial plexus. Proceedings of the Royal Society of Medicine, 51: 365-367.

Bonney, G., Birch, R., Jamieson, A. M. and Eames, R. A. (1984). Experience with vascularised nerve grafts. Clinics in Plastic Surgery, 11: 137-142.

Jones, S. J., Wynn Parry, C. B. and Landi, A. (1981). Diagnosis of brachial plexus traction lesions by sensory nerve action potentials and somatosensory evoked potentials. Injury, 12: 376–382.

Marshall, R. W. and De Silva, D. (in press). A study of CT contrast enhancement and cervical myelography in diagnosis of traction lesion of brachial plexus. Journal of Bone and Joint Surgery.

Narakas, A. (1978). Surgical treatment of traction injuries of the brachial plexus. Clinical Orthopaedics and Related Research, 133: 71–90.

Platt, H. (1921). The surgery of peripheral nerve injuries of warfare. British Medical Journal, 1: 596–600.

Platt, H. (1973). Obstetrical paralysis: A vanishing chapter in orthopaedic surgery. The Bulletin of the Hospital for Joint Diseases, 34: 4–21.

Wynn Parry, C. B. (1981). Rehabilitation of the hand (Fourth edition). London: Butterworth.

# 29

# INTERCOSTAL NERVE CROSSING AS A TREATMENT OF IRREPARABLY DAMAGED WHOLE BRACHIAL PLEXUS

N. Tsuyama
T. Hara
A. Nagano

## INTRODUCTION

Nerve crossing between the intercostal nerve and the musculocutaneous nerve was first attempted by Seddon (1963) with the intention of reinnervating the elbow flexor in patients with complete brachial plexus injury. He used the ulnar nerve as a free graft, and reported on one case. The number of brachial plexus injuries has increased rapidly in Japan, and since 1965 we have used our modification of this surgical procedure in patients with irreparably damaged whole brachial plexus (Tsuyama and Hara 1972a).

## PATIENTS AND METHODS

### Procedure

The third and fourth and at times fifth intercostal nerves were explored from the axilla to the tip of the rib, over as long a distance as possible, and usually about 12 cm. Temporary subperiosteal transection and retraction of the ribs facilitated the exposure of the nerve which ran between the periosteum and pleura. Utmost care was taken not to damage the pleura and intraoperative electrical stimulation was used to confirm the motor response of the abdominal muscles.

The distal ends of two or three nerves were severed, lined up and made into a cable by epineural suture. This cable was turned back, passed through the axilla to the upper arm and anastomosed to the musculocutaneous nerve as near as possible to its motor point in the biceps muscle, to shorten the distance the regenerating fibres must grow (Figure 1).

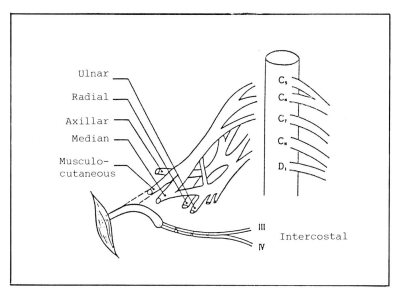

FIG. 1. Diagram showing the "anastomosis" of the 3rd and 4th intercostal nerves to the musculo-cutaneous nerve.

No nerve graft was used. The end of the cable was cut so that it was pointed like a pencil, the musculocutaneous nerve was cut in a 'V' shape to receive and wrap around the pointed end of the intercostal nerve cable. The shoulder was adducted to approximate the thin intercostal nerve cable and the thick musculocutaneous nerve which were sutured using a microsurgical technique of epineural suture with an atraumatic corneal needle.

Indications

This type of nerve crossing was only indicated in patients with root avulsion of the complete brachial plexus, in whom there was neither hope of spontaneous recovery nor of reconstruction, and the only other possibility of functional improvement had been amputation and prosthetic replacement. Therefore, an accurate diagnosis of root avulsion was important. Until 1980 root avulsion had been diagnosed by a combination of myelography, paralysis of the nerves which branch close to the roots, a positive Horner's sign, sensory and motor denervation in the area innervated by dorsal branch of the spinal nerves, a positive axon reflex such as the histamine flare test and positive detection of the evoked sensory nerve action potential in the area with complete sensory loss (Tsuyama and Hara 1972b, Nagano et al.

1984).    Recently  myelography using water soluble radioopaque dye with
CT scanning has been found to be very useful.

Since 1981 it has become our routine to explore all the patients  and
the level of the nerve damage was confirmed not only macroscopically but
also by somatosensory evoked cerebral cortical potential by  stimulating
intraoperatively  the  individual  root  outlets  (Sugioka  et al. 1982,
Sugioka 1984).  A negative somatosensory  evoked  EEG  and  a  positive
evoked  peripheral  sensory nerve action potential was definite evidence
of preganglionic i.e. root avulsion injury.   When the irreparability of
the lesion had been confirmed the intercostal nerve crossing was carried
out.

Assessment

In successful cases, volitional small  action  potentials  synchronizing
with  respiratory  movement began to appear in the electromyogram of the
biceps muscle 6 to 8 months postoperatively and these action  potentials
gradually  developed  into  an  interference  pattern,  and  voluntary
contraction  and  control  of  the  elbow  flexor  developed,  showing
sufficient endurance (Figures 2 and 3).

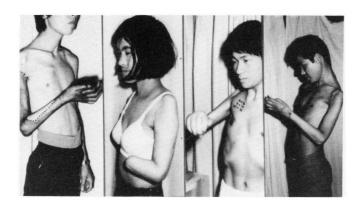

FIG.  2.  Clinical  results  of intercostal nerve crossing resulting in
active elbow flexion against gravity.

At the initial  stage  of  recovery,  when  the  patient  sneezed  or
coughed, involuntary elbow flexion occurred;  and the interval variation
diagram of the repetition of a  single  motor  unit  discharge  in  the
electromyogram  showed a clear respiratory rhythm.   However, within 18

to 24 months, patients could suppress this involuntary respiratory
component and learn to maintain elbow flexion with good voluntary
control.    This shows the separation of the voluntary and involuntary
components of the respiratory function, in other words, plasticity of
the nervous system.

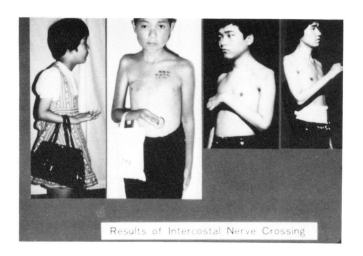

FIG. 3. Clinical results.    Patients may have sufficient control of
elbow flexion to allow them to carry bags on their forearm.

Further Treatment
In patients with good recovery of elbow flexion, the shoulder was  fused
in 20° abduction, so that the patient could adduct the arm by
contracting the middle part of the trapezius and could hold things under
his axilla.    For this reason we never used the accessory nerve.
Sensory recovery in the area of the lateral antebrachial cutaneous nerve
was also seen, although sensory switching was poor.

   To overcome the supinated position of the hand, the biceps tendon
could be rerouted and converted to an active pronator according to
Owing-Zancolli's procedure.    The wrist joint was sometimes also fused.


RESULTS


The following criteria were used to evaluate the results.    Elbow flexor
power of more than 4 was classified as excellent, 3 to 4 as good, 1 to 2
as fair and 0 as poor.

Intercostal nerve crossing to the musculocutaneous nerve was carried out in 156 patients between 1965 and 1985, of which 116 were followed up for more than 18 months. The average follow-up period was 5·7 years. The age of the patients at the time of surgery ranged from 3 years to 50 years and 89·7% of them were in their second or third decades. The majority of patients were operated upon within 6 months of the injury, but 30 patients (26·3%) underwent surgery more than 6 months after the injury.

Excellent results were obtained in 35 patients (30·2%), good in 42 (36·2%) and fair or poor in 39 patients (33·6%). Seventy-seven (66·4%) of the 116 operated cases could flex their elbow joints at least against gravity.

The results were better in those patients who underwent operation within 6 months of the injury and in the younger patients. The results were much poorer in patients more than 31 years of age.

## DISCUSSION

Our results indicate that intercostal nerve crossing to the musculocutaneous nerve is useful in many younger patients with an irreparably damaged entire brachial plexus which previously was considered to have a hopeless prognosis.

As a result of this study we now carry out free muscle transplants with a neurovascular pedicle which is anastomosed to the intercostal nerve cable and local vessels in patients who present late or are older.

## REFERENCES

Nagano, A., Tsuyama, N., Hara, T., and Sugioka, H. (1984). Brachial plexus injuries. Prognosis of postganglionic lesions. Archives of Orthopaedic and Traumatic Surgery, 102: 172-178.

Seddon, H. J. (1963). Nerve grafting. Journal of Bone and Joint Surgery, 45-B: 447-461.

Sugioka, H. (1984). Evoked potentials in the investigation of traumatic

lesions of the peripheral nerve and brachial plexus. Clinical
Orthopaedics and Related Research, 184:  85-92.

Sugioka, H., Tsuyama, N., Hara, T., Nagano, A., Tachibana, S. and
Ochiai, N. (1982). Investigation of brachial plexus injuries by
intraoperative cortical somatosensory evoked potentials. Archives of
Orthopaedic and Traumatic Surgery, 99:  143-151.

Tsuyama, N. and Hara, T. (1972a). Intercostal nerve transfer in the
treatment of brachial plexus injury of root-avulsion type. Proceedings
of the 12th Congress of SICOT, Tel Aviv, 1972, Excerpta Medica,
Amsterdam, p. 351.

Tsuyama, N. and Hara, T. (1972b). Diagnosis and treatment of brachial
plexus injury. Proceedings of the 12th Congress of SICOT, Tel Aviv,
1972, Excerpta Medica, Amsterdam, p. 504.

# 30. THE ANTERIOR APPROACH TO THE DISLOCATED SACROILIAC JOINT. REDUCTION AND FIXATION WITH A SQUARE PLATE.

S. Olerud
M. Hamberg

## INTRODUCTION

The sacro-iliac joint is dislocated in about 25% of unstable pelvic ring fractures. The injury is usually of high velocity such as a road traffic accident or a fall from height. An antero-posterior compression injury, a sheering force and even a lateral compression injury may be causative. In 7% of patients both sacro-iliac joints are involved. Major soft tissue injuries often also occur.

A dislocated sacro-iliac joint always indicates a major instability between the ilium and the sacrum. The very strong posterior ligaments are ruptured, as well as the sacrospinous ligament. The rather weak anterior sacro-iliac ligaments are of no importance in this context.

A dislocated sacro-iliac joint seems to be a major cause of late sequelae to pelvic injuries resulting in back pain and unequal limb lengths. Fifty per cent of the patients with this injury have a permanent disability.

The present treatment of these injuries varies a great deal. Wilson suggested femoral traction in combination with a pelvic sling (Wilson 1982). This requires prolonged bed rest, with unpredictable results.

External fixation, an excellent method for the open book injuries, where the posterior ligamentous structures are intact, has been tested many times with different configurations of external devices of varying complexity. The compression effect on a dislocated sacro-iliac joint only displaces the joint further as there are no intact structures to stabilise the joint. Tile (1984) suggested a combination of external fixation with femoral traction to counteract the sacro-iliac dislocation. The patient is confined to the bed for a considerable time with this treatment. The trend today is to stabilise the pelvis in such a way that it is easy to care for the patient, and to mobilise him out of bed as soon as possible. Internal fixation is very attractive, provided it can be done in a safe and a simple way.

Internal fixation from a posterior approach has some drawbacks. The position for the patient during surgery (lateral or prone) is cumbersome and may be difficult in patients who are seriously injured. The reduction of the joint may be complicated and can only be checked indirectly by palpation with the index finger which needs to pass under the sacro-iliac joint to the inner side of the pelvis.

A major disadvantage with the posterior approach may be the skin and muscles, which often have been traumatized in the injury. As a result skin healing may be affected and skin necrosis develop.

Since 1981 we have used an anterior approach very similar to that described by Avila (1941) for infections around the sacro-iliac joint.

## SURGICAL TECHNIQUE

The patient is placed in a supine position and each leg is individually draped. It should be possible to flex the hip on the injured side to 90° during the operation as well as adduct it. The incision follows the iliac crest, and is extended beyond the anterior iliac spine for a further 4-5 cm. in the line of the inguinal ligament. The abdominal muscles are sharply dissected medially from the iliac crest which is followed anteriorly to just below the anterior iliac spine. The lateral cutaneous nerve of the thigh is identified and freed cranially as well as caudally for about 4-5 cm. in both directions. The iliac crest is followed posteriorly. The inner table of the ilium is exposed subperiostally and the sacro-iliac joint displayed. The dissection continues subperiostally along the sacrum for a further 15 mm. The L4 and L5 nerves lie in front of the periosteum and will not be seen. During this dissection, the hip joint should be flexed to 90° and adducted, diminishing the tension of the nerves and psoas muscle. Two or three 3 mm. K-wires, 300 mm. long, are then hammered into the sacrum to hold the soft tissues medially during the rest of the operation.

The sacro-iliac joint can now be inspected, and debris in the joint space is removed. Often there are a number of loose pieces of cartilage, which otherwise would have affected bone union. By manipulating the loose ilium, the sacro-iliac joint can be reduced under vision to an anatomical position and a temporary pin is passed percutaneously through the ilium and across the sacro-iliac joint for 1 to 2 cm.   The pin can easily be observed passing from the iliac side of the sacro-iliac joint across the joint and into the sacrum.

A difficult reduction may be due to other pelvic fractures, which have to be exposed to facilitate reduction.   This complementary surgery is easily carried out with the patient on his back.   A distractor may be used to manipulate and reduce the other fractures and in difficult cases it is possible to fix one half of the pelvis to the table.

The fixation of the sacro-iliac joint is carried out with a special plate - which is square with two oval, elongated holes, allowing the surgeon to place two screws very close to each other and into the subchondral bone on each side of the sacro-iliac joint.   This gives the possibility of applying compression across the joint.   With cancellous bone graft in the joint space the chances for bone healing are excellent.

The position of the plate is shown in Figure 1.   In the wound the screws are easily reached with an ordinary screw driver.   Once in place, the sacro-iliac joint is completely locked, the temporary pin is removed and the operation completed.

To allow immediate mobilization with crutches we advocate complementary external fixation with a single bar attached to 6 mm. bone screws inserted just above the anterior inferior iliac spine (just above the origin of the rectus femoris).   The external fixation is maintained for 2-3 months.

The square plate has been tested biomechanically by Berner (1985) and is superior to posterior fixation with two screws and similar to two screws and a plate.

RESULTS

Fifteen patients have been followed for at least a year.   There were 11 men and 4 women with an age distribution of 18-45 years.   Eleven of the 15 injuries were due to traffic accidents.

Nine patients had further fractures of their pelvic ring, one patient had a bilateral dislocation and one had a fracture-dislocation on the

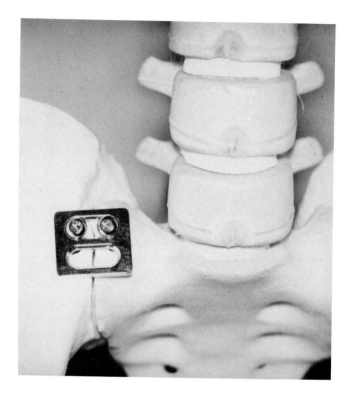

FIG. 1.    The square plate mounted on the pelvis.    Two screws in the
upper hole of the plate give compression of the sacro-iliac  joint  when
driven  home.    The fixation is completed by attaching two screws in the
lower hole, controlling rotatory stability.    All the screws should pass
into the subchondral bone on each side of the sacro-iliac joint.

contralateral side.

Thirteen  sacro-iliac  joints  were  completely reduced, and two with
less than $\frac{1}{2}$ cm. separation.   Most  of  the  other  ring  fractures  were
reduced  and  internally  fixed.     All concomitant acetabular fractures
were congruently reduced.

Six of the 15 injured patients had primary neurological defects.    Of
these,  3  recovered  completely  and  3  have  permanent peroneal nerve
paresis.

All 15 patients had healed clinically and radiographically at a  year
but  one  patient  required  revision  after  5  months  because  of  a
pseudarthrosis at the sacro-iliac joint.    The same  approach  was  used
including bone grafting into the joint space.

None  of  the  patients  developed disabling sacro-iliac pain but two
complained of back fatigue.

The leg lengths were equal in 13 of the 15 patients.

## Illustrative case report

A 35-year old lady was run over by a truck which resulted in a bilateral sacro-iliac joint dislocation (Figure 2a).    She was treated initially with an external fixator but the dislocation became more pronounced.  A month after the accident she was referred to our hospital where she was treated with an anterior bilateral approach and reduction of both dislocated sacro-iliac joints.   These were both fixed with the square plate but a separation less than 5 mm. wide had to be left on the left (Figure 2b).   Mobilization was started after 8 weeks with progressively increasing weight bearing.   Since her fourteenth post-operative week the lady has been completely free from disability and pain (Figure 2c).

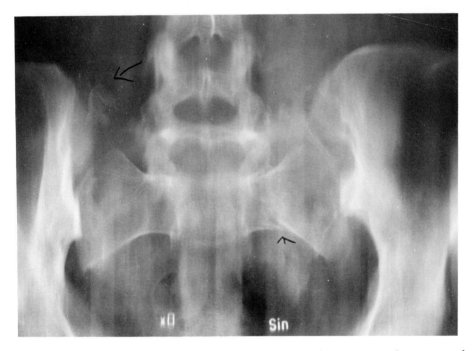

FIG. 2(a).    Bilateral sacro-iliac joint dislocation and a sacral fracture 30 days after a road traffic accident.


## CONCLUSIONS


The advantages of the square plate and 'he anterior approach are:-

    (i)    A supine patient at surgery which often is of value in multi-injured patients.

(ii)   A complete reduction can usually and easily be done under
       visual control.

(iii)  There is a small risk of soft tissue complications, since the
       incision does not involve areas on which the patient lies.

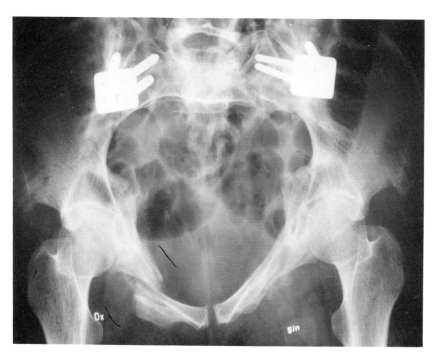

FIG. 2(b).   Inlet view of the pelvis after reduction and fixation  with
square   plate   on   each   side.    Anatomical  reduction  of  the   right
sacro-iliac joint has been achieved.   On the  left  there  is  a  minor
residual separation probably because of the sacral fracture.


REFERENCES


Avila, L. (1941).   Primary  pyogenic  infection  of  the  sacro-iliac
articulation.  A new approach to the  joint.   Report  of  seven  cases.
Journal of Bone and Joint Surgery, 23:  922-928.


Berner, W. (1985).  Personal communication.


Tile, M. (1984).   Fractures of the pelvis and acetabulum.   Williams and
Wilkins, Baltimore.

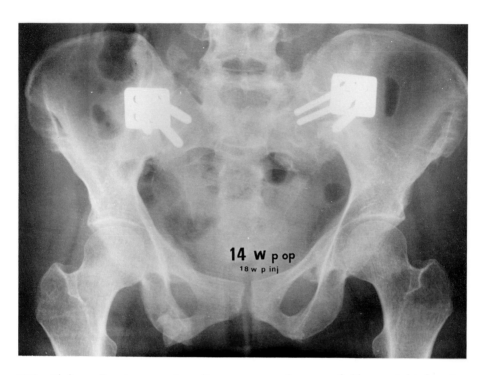

FIG. 2(c). Fourteen weeks after surgery she was fully weight-bearing and six months later the patient was completely rehabilitated without any sign of disability.

Wilson, J. N. (1982). Treatment of disruptions of the pelvic ring. In: Watson-Jones Fractures and Joint Injuries, 2nd Edition. (Ed. Wilson, J. N.), Churchill Livingstone, Edinburgh, London, New York, pp. 862-866.

## 31. THE TREATMENT OF NON-UNION

L. Read
M. Arafa
C. S. B. Galasko

### INTRODUCTION

Fracture treatment is always attended by a small incidence of non-union whether that treatment be conservative or surgical. Healing of an acute fracture or of bone following a surgical procedure can be affected by many factors: the degree of soft tissue injury, comminution, distraction, displacement, hormonal factors, electrical factors and the presence of infection. Often related to these are the two most basic factors – movement of the bony fragments and the local blood supply. Conventional methods of treatment of non-union address these two main factors, conservatively by external cast immobilization and encouragement of physiological loading and muscle activity, and surgically by fixation and bone grafting techniques. Proponents of the various methods described report success rates between 80% and 100% (Boyd et al. 1965, Weber and Cech 1976). However, these reports are of series of selected cases and a single method does not answer the needs of every patient with a non-union.

More recently it has been reported that electrical stimulation of bone will remove the need for operative treatment but, again, these are reports of selected cases.

### PATIENTS AND METHODS

One hundred and thirty consecutive patients (76 male, 54 female) referred to the non-union clinic of the University of Manchester Department of Orthopaedic Surgery have been studied in order to gain an overall picture of the problems associated with non-union; to assess the success of a variety of treatment methods including that of direct current stimulation, and to determine whether the addition of direct current stimulation to a conventional method increased its success rate.

The patients, for the most part, had been referred after failure of an initial or several attempts to obtain union. The average age was 37·8 years (range 15 years to 83 years) and the average time since injury was 17·5 months (range 5 months to 13 years). Fifty five per cent had had an open fracture, 45% had been comminuted, 55% had had at least one previous operation and 29% were, or had been, infected.

Fifteen of the 130 patients continued with the treatment undertaken before referral or declined the treatment advised. Each of the remaining 115 patients, 60% of whom were more than 9 months since injury, was allocated to one of 4 groups.

Group 1

Group 1 consisted of 45 patients who did not require operation for any of a number of factors commonly associated with non-union. Malalignment or displacement would require operative correction before the non-union could be tackled. A gap greater than 0·5 cm or excessive mobility (indicating the presence of synovium-lined cyst between the bone ends) would also be an indication for operative treatment, as would the presence of deep infection with necrotic, infected bone and soft tissue. In some patients an inappropriately sited implant or intact fibula splinted the fracture apart and in others a broken, loose implant complicated the picture. The 45 patients in Group 1 had a well aligned bone, a gap less than 0·5 cm, no distracting or broken implant and no significant infection. These patients were treated by a period of continuous direct current stimulation while the limb was immobilised in a cast. The other 70 patients (60·9%) had one or more of the above features associated with their non-union.

There were 36 tibial and 4 femoral non-unions, 3 instances of failed arthrodesis of the knee and 2 forearm non-unions in Group 1. The cathode (a Teflon-coated Kirschner wire) was passed into the distal fragment as close as possible to the fracture gap (under x-ray control) and the large anode strapped to the skin proximally. The limb was immobilised in a cast, or spica and patients with lower limb non-unions were instructed not to bear weight on the affected side. The stimulation was maintained for an average of 10·7 weeks (range 6 to 20 weeks), and the patient then allowed to weight bear in a protective cast until clinical union was achieved. The clinical decision regarding union was proven subsequently by radiographic demonstration of cortical continuity and remedullarisation after several more months of remodelling had occurred.

## Group 2

Thirty one patients, comparable to those in other groups, comprised Group 2. They underwent a conventional operation such as Phemister bone grafting with or without internal or external fixation. The first part of the operation was designed to deal with the particular factor associated with the non-union: 4 of the 14 tibial non-unions underwent a modified Papineau technique and 2 of the 15 femoral cases had a two-stage procedure for gross infection. There were 2 forearm bone non-unions treated by plating and grafting. None of these patients had their non-union electrically stimulated.

## Group 3

To test the hypothesis that direct current stimulation could be used to advantage in the immediate post operative period a comparable group of 28 patients had direct current stimulation added for 12 weeks following a conventional operation. There were 11 tibial non-unions, 4 failed arthrodeses and 6 others.

## Group 4

A small group of 9 patients (Group 4) presented with atrophy and non-union around a secure implant. Instead of further bone grafting, direct current stimulation was given for 12 weeks without disturbing the fixation. There were 3 plated tibiae, 3 femora with a Küntscher nail and 3 femora with a Huckstep nail.

## RESULTS

The results of the patients in Group 1 are shown in Table 1. Thirty of the 36 tibial non-unions united, a success rate of 83·3%: one successful case required later curettage for a localised area of bone infection. Only 1 of 4 femoral non-unions immobilised in a spica and

stimulated  for  a period of up to 20 weeks healed (25%) and none of the
3 failed arthrodeses responded to stimulation while in a cylinder cast.

## TABLE 1

The  infection  and  success  rates in patients receiving direct current
stimulation - Group 1.

| Site of non-union | Number | Developed Infection | United | % Success |
|---|---|---|---|---|
| Tibia | 36 | 1 | 30 | 83·3 |
| Femur | 4 | 0 | 1 | 25 |
| Arthrodesis | 3 | 0 | 0 | 0 |
| Other | 2 | 0 | 2 | 100 |
| TOTAL | 45 | 1 | 33 | 73·3 |

The overall success rate in Group 2 (who did not  receive  electrical
stimulation) was 83·7% with the tibial fractures having a higher rate of
union (92·8%) than the femoral non-unions (73·3%) (Table 2).

## TABLE 2

The infection and  success  rates  in  patients  receiving  conventional
operative treatment - Group 2.

| Site of non-union | Number | Developed Infection | United | % Success |
|---|---|---|---|---|
| Tibia | 14 | 2 | 13 | 92·8 |
| Femur | 15 | 0 | 11 | 73·3 |
| Other | 2 | 0 | 2 | 100 |
| TOTAL | 31 | 2 | 26 | 83·7 |

The  results  of the patients in Group 3 (conventional operation plus
electrical stimulation) is shown in Table  3.    There  was  a  marginal
overall  improvement over Group 2 (87%) but the numbers and diversity of
associated factors do not permit of statistical analysis.

TABLE 3

The infection and success rates in patients receiving conventional
operative treatment with post operative direct current stimulation –
Group 3.

| Site of non–union | Number | Developed Infection | United | % Success |
|---|---|---|---|---|
| Tibia | 11 | 0 | 10 | 90·9 |
| Femur | 7 | 0 | 7 | 100 |
| Arthrodesis | 4 | 0 | 3 | 75 |
| Other | 6 | 0 | 5 | 83 |
| TOTAL | 28 | 0 | 25 | 89 |

The overall results in Group 4 were disappointing (Table 4) with only
44% success:   only  the  less rigid Küntscher femoral nail allowed new
bone to form across the gap.   Operation in the form of further grafting
appears  preferable  in  these particular cases and should be offered to
the patient before the implant breaks.

TABLE 4

The infection and success rates in  patients  receiving  direct  current
stimulation with a rigid implant in situ – Group 4.

| Site of non–union | Number | Developed Infection | United | % Success |
|---|---|---|---|---|
| Tibia | 3 | 1 | 1 | 33 |
| Femur – Küntscher nail | 3 | 0 | 3 | 100 |
| Femur – Huckstep nail | 3 | 0 | 0 | 0 |
| TOTAL | 9 | 1 | 4 | 44 |

CONCLUSION

Our  results  suggest  that  60%  of  non-unions will  require surgery to
achieve control of  associated  factors  such  as  malalignment,  a  gap

greater than 0·5 cm, excessive mobility, deep infection, broken implant, intact fibula splinting the fracture ends apart, and atrophic non-union around a secure implant; but in carefully selected cases of tibial, radial and ulnar non-union there is an 85-90% chance of union with direct current stimulation, immobilisation and non weight bearing. The hypothesis that direct current stimulation during the post operative period may augment bone healing after conventional operation requires further investigation.

## REFERENCES

Boyd, H. B., Anderson, L. D. and Johnston, D. S. (1965). Changing concepts in the treatment of non-union. Clinical Orthopaedics and Related Research, 43: 37-54.

Weber, B. G. and Cech, O. (1976). Pseudarthrosis. Hans Huber Medical Publisher, Berne, Switzerland.

# 32.THE LEEDS-KEIO LIGAMENT IN CHRONIC ANTERIOR CRUCIATE DEFICIENCY

S. J. McLoughlin
R. B. Smith

## INTRODUCTION

Ligament reconstruction in the knee is undergoing a period of innovation and re-appraisal.  Well established techniques using  local  autogenous tissues  are  being  re-assessed  in  view  of  their  often complicated procedures, inevitable damage to 'normal' structures  and  mechanisms, difficulties  in  fixation  and  somewhat  variable  long  term  results (Johnson et al. 1984, Paterson and Trickey, 1986).

Carbon fibre unfortunately, has not lived up to initial  expectations and  polyester  based  prostheses  have been developed independently, in several centres (Rushton  et  al.  1983).   This  prosthesis  and  the technique of insertion was designed and developed at Leeds University by Dr. B. B. Seedhom and Dr. K. Fujikawa,  visiting  research  fellow  from Keio University, Tokyo.

## MATERIAL, PATIENTS AND METHODS

The  polyester  ligament  takes  the  form  of  an  open  weave tube one centimetre in diameter, open at each end to take the insertion of  bone plugs which eventually produce biological anchoring of the prosthesis by bony ingrowth through the open weave.  The strength of  the  prosthesis is similar to that of the natural anterior cruciate ligament and testing by  prolonged  cyclical  loading  has  confirmed  its  durability  under repeated stress.

The  technique,  used  in  this  series  was  one  of intra-articular replacement of the anterior cruciate ligament alone,  using  simple  but well  designed  instrumentation.   The instruments consist of a 'G' clamp jig, bone plug reamer, bone plug extractor, 6·3 mm drill and guide sleeve and a bone plug punch.

## Surgical technique

An extended medial parapatellar incision was used to gain good exposure of the lateral femoral condyle and upper, medial border of the tibia; smaller separate femoral and tibial incisions can be made if preferred.

Accurate placement and sound fixation of the jig was essential. Bone plugs were cut from the femur and tibia, and using the guide sleeve the tunnels were drilled. The ligament was passed through the tibial and femoral tunnels, the femoral bone plug inserted and with the knee flexed to approximately 30° maximal tension was applied to the ligament before inserting the tibial bone plug. For added security a staple was applied to both the femoral and tibial ends of the ligament. If placement had been accurate, the intra-articular portion of the ligament was isometric when the knee was flexed and extended.

After wound closure the knee was immobilised in a full leg plaster with the knee flexed approximately 30°. After two weeks, the plaster was changed and the sutures removed. At six weeks a hinged brace was applied allowing flexion/extension movements from 10 to 90°. Physiotherapy was started from day one with static quadriceps exercises but after removal of the brace a much more aggressive regimen was started.

## Clinical indications

The indication for surgery in this series was chronic anterior cruciate ligament insufficiency leading to instability and giving way of the affected knee on walking or light sporting activity. All patients had a significant anterior drawer sign and almost all patients had a positive pivot shift or jerk test pre-operatively. All patients underwent intensive physiotherapy prior to being considered for surgery and an examination under anaesthetic and arthroscopy was carried out in all cases.

## RESULTS

The results from four centres (Preston, Harrogate, Bradford and Hull) have been combined and the first 50 patients have been assessed. Forty-one were male and 9 female.  Their ages ranged from 18 to 47 with a mean of 27 years.  All patients complained of giving way and many of pain and swelling.

The causal injury was as follows:  football (22), rugby (9), squash (3), skiing (2), road traffic accidents (6), fall (7) and cricket (1). Fifteen patients had had previous meniscal surgery and at the time of ligament replacement a further 7 had evidence of meniscal pathology, requiring partial or total meniscectomy.  Five patients had medial capsular laxity repaired, in the main by pes anserinus transfer.  The follow-up ranged from 9 months to $3\frac{1}{2}$ years.

Pre-operatively all patients had 2+ or 3+ anterior draw with the knee examined at 30°.  Post-operatively 32 patients had their anterior laxity eliminated, but 28 patients retained a lesser degree of anterior draw.

Pre-operatively all the patients had a 2+ or 3+ anterior draw at 90°. Post-operatively 22 patients had no anterior draw whilst 28 retained some degree of anterior movement.

The jerk test was eliminated in almost all patients, having been positive in all pre-operatively.  Post-operatively only 3 patients demonstrated this instability.

Subjective evaluation of the operation was made using the Cincinatti sports medicine assessment grading.  This is a self assessment rating filled in by the patient, with a maximum score of 100.  Pain (20), swelling (10), giving way (20), function, work and sport (20) and exercise performance – walking (10), stairs (10), running (5), jumping or twisting activities (5) are assessed.

The overall mean improvement was from 35% pre-operatively to 77% post-operatively.

A score 75% and above was classified as 'good', between 50 and 75% as fair and a score under 50% as poor.  The following results were obtained:

| | | |
|---|---|---|
| (75% plus) | Good – considerable improvement | 38 patients |
| (50–75% ) | Fair – some improvement | 10 patients |
| (<50% ) | Poor – no improvement | 2 patients. |

The average range of flexion at 9 months was 130° but this improved considerably by 18 months.

Arthroscopic review confirmed a clear coating of fibrous tissue and synovium surrounding the intra-articular portion of the implanted ligament and stained sections confirmed fibrous and bony ingrowth around the polyester weave in the bony tunnels.

## Complications

Complications included infection in one case. This was treated by continuous irrigation and settled without the prosthesis being removed. The patient is now playing competitive squash.

There were 2 cases of prosthetic loosening following trauma, 1 has been revised and revision is planned in the other patient. Both of these occurred at an early stage and were due to slippage of the ligament in the bony tunnels presumably before fibro-osseous ingrowth had occurred. In view of this all ligaments now have supplementary staple fixation to allow early mobilisation.

Three patients suffered patello-femoral pain. One had chondromalacia pre-operatively which became more troublesome after ligament insertion and a patella re-alignment procedure was successfully carried out.

## DISCUSSION

Fifty patients from the orthopaedic practice of 4 surgeons were reviewed. The overall results of the Leeds-Keio ligament for chronic anterior cruciate deficiency have been very acceptable, the vast majority of patients being pleased with the results of their surgery. Some patients have returned to professional sport but many have chosen not to subject their knees to the risk of further damage and now limit their sport to leisure.

Although a degree of laxity persisted in a proportion of the knees, it seemed that the patients found the elimination of a pivot shift or jerk was a major improvement.

'Long' ligaments with an antero-lateral component superficial to the lateral collateral ligament are now used more frequently, proving beneficial in patients with marked antero-lateral instability, and the basic technique discussed in this article has been extended for use in acute multi-ligament ruptures and posterior cruciate and collateral ligament reconstruction.

## REFERENCES

Johnson, R. J., Eriksonn, E., Haggmark, T. and Pope, M. H. (1984). Five to ten year follow-up evaluation after reconstruction of the anterior cruciate ligament. Clinical Orthopaedics and Related Research, 183: 122-140.

Paterson, F. W. N. and Trickey, E. L. (1986). Anterior cruciate ligament reconstruction using part of the patellar tendon as a free graft. Journal of Bone and Joint Surgery, 68-B: 453-457.

Rushton, N., Dandy, D. J. and Naylor, C. P. E. (1983). The clinical, arthroscopic and histological findings after replacement of the anterior cruciate ligament with carbon fibre. Journal of Bone and Joint Surgery, 65-B: 308-309.

# 33

POSTERIOR SEGMENTAL WIRING FOR SPINAL DEFORMITY:   THE HARTSHILL SYSTEM

J. Dove

## INTRODUCTION

Posterior segmental wiring of the spine is not a new concept.    In  the
1950's in Spain correction of spinal deformity was being performed using
tibial grafts segmentally wired to the base  of  the  spinous  processes
(Hernandez-Ros and Codorniu 1965).    At about the same time in Portugal,
Drs. Resina and Alves were developing a similar system using a malleable
metal rod (Resina 1963;   Resina and Ferreira Alves 1977).

It  was not, however, until the work of Dr. Luque in Mexico City that
posterior segmental wiring of the spine became internationally  popular.
Dr.   Luque  showed  that  sublaminar  wiring  was  a  very  strong  and
technically feasible means of correcting spinal deformity.    As a result
of  his  work, for many spinal surgeons throughout the world, sublaminar
wiring is the method of  choice  for  the  correction  of  neuromuscular
scoliosis (Luque 1974;   Luque 1984).

Dr. Luque's system involved the use of two 5 mm. stainless steel rods
with a right angle bent at each end and wired at each level to the spine
using a single loop of 1·2 mm. in diameter stainless steel wire.

The original Luque system has a number of disadvantages.    First, and
perhaps most important, even with experience it  is  very  difficult  to
obtain  secure  fixation  of the point where the rods overlap.    This is
essential, because if the fixation should come adrift, the rods are free
to  rotate  with  a  resultant  loss in correction of the deformity.    A
further problem with two separate  rods  is  that  when  the  wires  are
tightened  the  rods  inevitably  come to lie together in the midline so
that there is a reasonable correction of the scoliosis but a  very  poor
correction of rotation.

Along  with  a  number  of  other workers we, therefore, began to move

towards a rectangular system. It is possible to bend a rectangle at
the time of surgery but this is technically awkward and because the
rectangle is unwelded the same problem applies as with two separate
rods; in other words on tightening the wires the two limbs of the
rectangle come together in the midline with a resultant poor control of
rotation. We, therefore, developed the Hartshill rectangle. This is
a welded rectangle made from a stainless steel rod. A 100° roof is
bent into the rectangle at each end which allows the rectangle to sit
snuggly against the spine and is also important in making sure that at
each end the wires slide down the shoulders to lie in the corners of the
rectangle thereby giving important control of rotation at each end of
the rectangle. This is particularly important in shorter rectangles.

The rectangles come in two sizes being made of 5 mm. or 6 mm.
stainless steel rod and are available in a variety of lengths from 2 to
45 cm. in 1 cm. increments. The system is available from A. W. Showell
(Surgicraft) Limited of Redditch, England.

Based on our biomechanical tests we prefer to use 2 loops of 0·9 mm.
cold worked stainless steel wire at each level (Dove et al. 1983). We
have shown that this type of wiring is stronger than the original Luque
system and, in addition, cold worked wire is stiffer than heat worked
wire and is technically easier to pass through the spinal canal because
it retains better the shape that one has bent into it.

With the addition of a few simple tools the Hartshill system has
become our routine method for the internal fixation of the spine. The
commonest indications are spinal deformity, low back pain, spinal
fractures, neck pain and spinal tumours.

The first 33 cases where we used the Hartshill system for spinal
deformity have been separately reported (Dove, in press).


## PATIENTS AND METHODS


### Basic surgical technique

The essential technique consists of a posterior midline subperiosteal
dissection of the spine. Over the length of the spine that is to be
stabilised the spinous processes and interspinous ligaments are removed.
At each level a small window is made in the ligamentum flavum so that
wires can be passed. A rectangle of appropriate size and length is

selected and contoured as necessary. Prior to the passage of the wires, the facet joints are removed and the fusion bed prepared. The chosen rectangle is then threaded onto the wires and held securely against the spine using the Hartshill pushers. The wires are then tightened using a jet twister and cut short leaving a 1 cm. length of twist which is given the final tighten by turning it down away from the overlying muscle in the direction of the original twist. The wound is then closed.

For routine mobile adolescent idiopathic scoliosis where a rectangle of less than 24 cm. is indicated, a 5 mm. calibre rectangle is satisfactory. For longer curves, for a larger patient or for spinal fractures and kyphosis a 6 mm. calibre rectangle should be used.

In scoliosis the wires are tightened from the bottom upwards working on the convexity first. In adolescent idiopathic scoliosis when the midthoracic transverse processes are large enough, the wires at the apex of the concavity are passed around the transverse processes and tightened last of all in order to provide an improved correction of rotation.

After surgery the patient can mobilise when comfortable and usually leaves hospital in 10 days without the need for any form of post-operative bracing for straightforward adolescent idiopathic scoliosis.

However, for kyphosis, for thoracolumbar fracture dislocations or in patients where I wish to mould the rib hump, I use a removable brace post-operatively.

## Synopsis of patients

The following is the breakdown of our first 100 patients treated for spinal deformity using the Hartshill system:

| | |
|---|---|
| Scoliosis | 38 patients |
| Kyphosis | 18 patients |
| Spinal fractures | 26 patients |
| Spondylolisthesis | 18 patients |
| Total = 100 patients | |

The age range of the patients was from 2 to 78 years with a follow-up of 1 to 4 years (mean 2·4 years).

## Complications

With any new system and in particular one that invades the spinal canal the question of the complications is an extremely important one.  There is no doubt that with segmental wiring attention to detail is important and particularly when used for spinal deformity it is not a system to be used by an "occasional" spinal surgeon.

The following complications have occurred:

| | |
|---|---|
| Broken wires | 7 patients |
| Infection | 2 patients |
| CSF leak | 2 patients |
| Neurological | 2 patients |

## Neurological complications

These merit further discussion.

The first case was a patient with an idiopathic scoliosis who developed a footdrop, the mechanism of which was unclear.  This resolved completely within six months.

The other patient posed a more important problem.  The patient probably had a juvenile idiopathic scoliosis and presented with a 130° curve and radiographic evidence of upper thoracic cord compression but no pre-operative neurological signs.  The first stage was an anterior decompression of the cord through a thoracotomy and was uneventful.  Three weeks later a posterior approach using the Hartshill system was performed after which the patient was permanently paraplegic.  I have carried out a morbidity study by questionnaire amongst members of the British Scoliosis Society in order to compare the morbidity of segmental spinal wiring with conventional methods.  That study showed that in the years 1983 and 1984 there were 16 serious neurological complications amongst a total of 1,121 operations for spinal deformity.  Eight of these occurred in cases where staged anterior and posterior surgery had been carried out and these were of course the cases with the most severe curves.  If one considers only the serious complications of complete or partial paraplegia and if one considers only the common condition of adolescent idiopathic scoliosis, then there were 4 cases of paraplegia; 3 in Harri-Luque's and 1 with Harrington instrumentation.  It was a conclusion of that study that the Harri-Luque system using a combination of segmental wires in combination with a Harrington distraction system is potentially dangerous (Dove 1985).


## CONCLUSION

The Hartshill system is an inexpensive and adaptable system that can be used for any type of spinal disorder and that can be used at any age throughout the spine from skull to sacrum. No expensive instrumentation is required. Attention to detail in the technique, especially for the surgery of deformity, is essential.


## REFERENCES

Dove, J. (1986). Segmental spinal instrumentation: British Scoliosis Society morbidity report. Journal of Bone and Joint Surgery, 68-B: 680.

Dove, J. (in press). Luque segmental spinal instrumentation: the use of the Hartshill rectangle. Orthopedics.

Dove, J., von Bottenburg, H., Arnold, P. and Ali, M. S. (1983). Biomechanical aspects of Luque segmental spinal instrumentation. Presented at the First European Congress on Scoliosis and Kyphosis, Dubrovnick.

Hernandez-Ros, A. and Codorniu (1965). Neuvas tactica y tecnica operatonias an al tratamiento & e las escoliosis. Scritti medici in onove ti P. del torto. Saveriu Pipola, Napoli, pp. 71-97.

Luque, E. R. (1974). Anatomy of scoliosis and its correction. Clinical Orthopaedics and Related Research, 105: 298.

Luque, E. R. (1984). Segmental spinal instrumentation: the state of the art. Slack, pp. 1-11.

Resina, J. (1963). Redressement et stabilisation immédiate des scoliosis par un tuteur métallique. Associatione Européene contre la

<u>Poliomyelite, IX Symposium, Stockholm.</u>  Masson  et  Cie,  Paris,  pp.
421–429.


Resina, J. and Ferreira Alves, A. (1977).  A technique of correction and
internal fixation for scoliosis.  <u>Journal of  Bone  and  Joint  Surgery,</u>
59–B:  159–165.

34.
# SIMULTANEOUS COMBINED ANTERIOR AND POSTERIOR FUSION:   A SURGICAL SOLUTION FOR FAILED SPINAL SURGERY

J. P. O'Brien

## INTRODUCTION

There is no field of clinical medicine more distressing than those patients who have been disabled following repeated operations for low back and leg pain.  The continuing failure of posterior surgery to relieve the patient of his pain renders him more disabled, unemployable and so distressed he is often suicidal.

It is against this background that Simultaneous Combined Anterior and Posterior Fusion has evolved, namely an attempt to rehabilitate this challenging group of people where conventional repeat operations have been shown to be futile (Waddell et al. 1979).

The concept of two operations in severe back pain became apparent following the established success of the combined approach to severe spinal deformities which emerged from Hong Kong in 1970 and later.  For example, in severe scoliosis, it became apparent that either anterior or posterior surgery alone would be likely to fail, whereas the combination of anterior correction and fusion by the Dwyer technique together with posterior fusion and Harrington instrumentation made excellent correction possible and a high fusion rate more certain (O'Brien and Yau 1972).  This combined approach, applicable to all severe fixed curvatures, has altered the entire management of the deformed spine.

## THE SIMULTANEOUS COMBINED ANTERIOR AND POSTERIOR FUSION (SCAPF)

### The Evolution
Anterior fusion alone for the treatment of the so-called post-laminectomy syndrome had a small but real incidence of

pseudarthrosis, especially when a large laminectomy defect existed. The inherent instability from such a laminectomy defect did not provide the necessary protection for the anterior grafts and these were submitted to excessive rocking, preventing vascularisation of the graft which led to possible delay in union and perhaps pseudarthrosis. This produced a significant delay in the rehabilitation of the patient and with a possibility of permanent disability (O'Brien et al. 1986).

Posterior fusion alone, even in the presence of internal fixation, had several drawbacks:

    (i)    The pain sensitive disc tissue was left in situ (Yoshizawa et al. 1980).

    (ii)   Posterior or lateral fusion, with or without internal fixation, was biomechanically inferior to anterior fusion. Both anterior and posterior fusions have been shown to be biomechanically inferior to the Simultaneous Combined Anterior and Posterior Fusion.

Each motion segment is really a three-joint complex involving a disc and two facet joints. The ideal from a mechanical point of view is to deal with all three joints and the simultaneous combined operation does precisely this.


Principles involved with the simultaneous combined procedure


    (i)    Correct the deformity within the motion segment.

Invariably there has been height loss with disc excision and it is an important principle that this deformity or height loss be corrected so as to enlarge the intervertebral foramen. By so doing, the emerging nerve roots are decompressed. It must be emphasised again that the height of the intervertebral foramen and its restoration to normal are crucial.


    (ii)   Nerve root decompression should only be carried out when indicated.

When nerve root decompression is indicated, it can easily be carried out at the time of the posterior instrumentation and fusion. If any doubt exists regarding the possible compression of the nerve roots, caution indicates that they must be inspected.

(iii) <u>Maintain the natural lumbar lordosis by performing the anterior fusion first</u>.

If this is not carried out, and posterior surgery performed with instrumentation, the natural lordosis will be flattened, leading to an unsightly iatrogenic deformity.  The lordosis can be increased by using strong distractors to open up the disc space before inserting a maximum volume of bone graft, usually a mixture of Cloward-type allograft (Cloward 1980) with autograft obtained by the so-called window technique through a separate incision from the left iliac crest.

(iv) <u>Posterior instrumention is important.</u>

Ideally this is a distraction form of instrumentation to ensure that the anterior grafts are locked firmly in compression.  The Knodt rods are ideal, simple though they may be;  the pedicular system also allows for distraction of the fusion segments which is an important principle in this technique.

## Indications

The precise indications for this major surgical reconstruction of the lumbar spine are still being developed.  However, there are two main broad groups:

(i)   Failed previous back surgery (the majority).

(ii)  Severely disabled patients without any previous surgery who have been disabled for a significant period of time, despite all forms of conservative treatment.

In the case of a heavily-built patient who is unemployed because of back pain, but could, if rehabilitated within a short period, take up employment again, it is essential to consider the SCAPF technique with its fast recuperative period and its positive solid fusion.

## Surgical procedure

In the first group of 35 patients, the combined procedure was carried out with the posterior fusion being done first, using double Harrington rods.  The patient was then turned most carefully and the standard retro-peritoneal anterior fusion followed.

In the second group, the order of the surgical procedure was reversed and the anterior fusion was done first, thus preserving most of the natural lordosis.  The preceding patients had lost their lordosis.

All procedures are now carried out with anterior surgery first, followed by posterior surgery with double Knodt rods.

There are several points of technical importance which should be emphasized:

(i)   Pre-operative planning:  this must include the number of levels to be fused front and back.   Two vertebrae are normally fused;  however, if the patient has already undergone many laminectomies at different levels, it is possible to fuse two levels anteriorly and four levels posteriorly.   The decision rests on the amount and extent of bone already removed from the spine during previous operations. Discography and tomography are invaluable and routine in the preliminary work-up.

(ii)  When the discs have been removed using the anterior retroperitoneal approach, strong distraction is used, and the maximum amount of autograft, supplemented by allograft, inserted into the interbody space.   This distraction of the interbody space decompresses the nerve roots by enlarging the intervertebral foramina (Figure 1).

(iii) The autograft is removed from the iliac crest by a separate incision (window technique).   The allograft is prepared using the Cloward dry method of preparation or frozen femoral head.

(iv)  Posterior instrumentation is essential to distract the motion segment and to compress the anterior grafts.   When the neural arches are intact and the instrumentation involves two levels, the Knodt rods are ideal for this purpose (Figure 2). However, multi-level laminectomies are better distracted and instrumented with double Harrington rods, which extend distally to the ala of the sacrum.   A careful technique of bilateral gutter fusion is essential, using a large volume of autograft. Simple facet joint arthodesis was not adequate in the first group of the series.

(v)   The main objection is the large amount of spinal surgery in one session.   It must be strongly emphasized that this technique demands an expert team, trained in both anterior and posterior spinal techniques.   This is vital as it ensures the speed and careful handling of tissues, which is very important to achieve a successful result and reduce the amount of

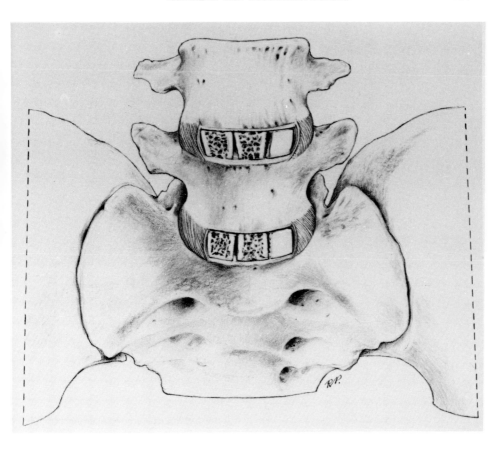

FIG. 1. Drawing of the front of the vertebral column to show the
anterior lumbar fusion technique. A minimum of three plugs are used to
replace the excised disc. Allograft will occasionally be required,
depending on the number of spaces to be fused. The main volume of bone
is removed from the left iliac crest.

operating time.

(vi) If, for some reason, the anterior surgery takes longer than an
acceptable length of time, posterior surgery should be delayed
for two weeks. This arrangement should always be clearly
explained to the patient undergoing the simultaneous combined
procedure before surgery is commenced.

The average time taken for the combined procedure was $3\frac{1}{4}$ hours and
the average blood loss was 600 mls. Post-operatively, the patients
were encouraged to stand within 48 hours and this was made possible by
the inherent stability of the motion segments following the combined
procedure. They were discharged from hospital 10-14 days after
surgery, wearing a light elasticized corset.

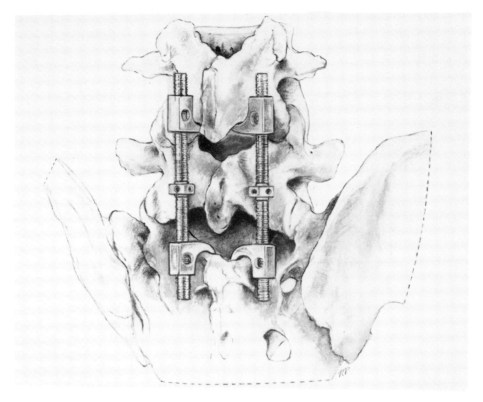

FIG. 2. Drawing of the posterior elements of the spine to demonstrate
the second stage of the combined anterior and posterior fusion. Double
Knodt rods in position between the lamina of L4 and the first sacral
arch. Finally, both bilateral gutters are decorticated and a large
volume of autograft mixed with allograft is packed into these recesses.


## DISCUSSION


It must be emphasized that this surgery is a major, new and radical
approach to the most difficult problem of the patient disabled following
repeated back surgery. This procedure must not be undertaken lightly
and the surgeon must be very experienced in the field of both anterior
and posterior spinal surgery before carrying out this major double
operation.

We have been constantly surprised at the incidence of tears in the
posterior annulus, as well as inflammatory changes in the anterior
annulus, seen in this group of disabled people (Jaffray and O'Brien
1986).

The most attractive features of this double procedure are that the pain-sensitive disc tissue is thoroughly removed, except for the remnants of posterior annulus, and inherent stability is provided with both the anterior grafts and with the posterior instrumentation and bilateral grafting. Removal of the instrumentation is only very occasionally required and is not resorted to as a routine measure.

Experience with over 200 patients over the past 6 years has indicated excellent to good results in over 80% of patients. It must be emphasized, however, that the principles detailed above must be clearly understood and adhered to if a high success rate is to be achieved.

## REFERENCES

Cloward, R. B. (1980). Gas sterilised cadaver bone grafts for spinal fusion operations: A simplified bone bank. Spine, 5: 4-10.

Jaffray, D. and O'Brien, J. P. (1986). Isolated intervertebral disc resorption - a source of mechanical and inflammatory back pain. Spine, 11: 397-401.

O'Brien, J. P. and Yau, A. C. M. C. (1972). Anterior and posterior correction and fusion for paralytic scoliosis. Clinical Orthopaedics and Related Research, 86: 151-153.

O'Brien, J. P., Dawson, M. H. O., Heard, C. W., Momberger, G., Speck, G. and Weatherley, C. R. (1986). Simultaneous combined anterior and posterior fusion - A surgical solution for failed spinal surgery with a brief review of the first 150 patients. Clinical Orthopaedics and Related Research, 203: 191-195.

Waddell, G., Kummel, E. G., Lotto, W. N., Graham, J. D., Hall, H. and McCulloch, J. A. (1979). Failed lumbar disc surgery and repeat surgery following industrial injuries. Journal of Bone and Joint Surgery, 61-A: 201-207.

Yoshizawa, H., O'Brien, J. P., Smith, W. T. and Trumper, M. (1980). The neuropathology of intervertebral discs removed for low back pain. Journal of Pathology, 132: 95-104.

## 35. CHRONIC INFLAMMATION IN MECHANICAL BACK PAIN SYNDROMES

M. I. V. Jayson

## INTRODUCTION

The traditional classification of the causes of back pain is divided into those arising from problems within the back and pain referred from elsewhere. Amongst the back problems are mechanical, inflammatory, neoplastic and metabolic disorders. The mechanical or structural problems are by far the most common and include prolapsed intervertebral disc and lumbar spondylosis. However, the mechanical model of pathogenesis of back pain fails to explain the characteristics that clinically are seen. In particular there is a poor correlation between radiographic evidence of lumbar spondylosis and the development of back pain (Lawrence 1977). The mechanical problem is persistent and long-lasting but the clinical character of this type of back pain is of acute episodes of pain and disability which usually resolve within a few days. It, therefore, appears that these mechanical and degenerative changes alone are not enough to account for the development of chronic back pain and other factors, presently poorly identified, must play an important role in the development of this problem. There is now evidence of secondary chronic inflammatory change occurring within the spine in many patients. This is of particular importance in patients with chronic persistent symptoms and the development of back pain is probably related to this.

## CHRONIC INFLAMMATION IN MECHANICAL PROBLEMS

Pathological examination of tissues surrounding a disc prolapse showed the presence of granulation tissue with chronic inflammatory changes

(Goldie, 1958, Hirsch 1959). Discs that prolapsed, and were painful
were at a lower pH than normal. This correlated with signs of
inflammation and scarring around the nerve roots (Diamant et al. 1968,
Nachemson 1969). Stimulation of a nerve root damaged by prolapse
produced pain, but stimulation of a nerve that had not previously been
damaged did not (Lindahl 1966). These studies implied that there were
important secondary changes occurring in the nerve root to produce the
response. Altered immunity has also been found in symptomatic disc
prolapse, again suggesting a degree of chronic inflammation (Bisla et
al. 1976).

## Arachnoiditis and nerve root sheath fibrosis

Scarring and thickening of the membranes surrounding the nerve roots
(arachnoiditis and nerve root sheath fibrosis) are recognised causes of
severe back pain and nerve root problems. The earliest reports
described these changes following previous infection, but they may also
occur following trauma and perhaps the use of spinal anaesthetics.
However, they develop most commonly in patients who have undergone
myelography using oil based media and/or who have undergone one or more
laminectomies (Burton 1978).

The diagnosis of arachnoiditis and nerve root sheath fibrosis is
difficult. Until recently, further myelography or radiculography was
required, but this type of investigation might be unwise in such
patients. The advent of CT scanning and MR imaging has enabled
recognition of these disorders in many difficult back pain problems.
However, the only definitive way of substantiating this diagnosis is by
histological analysis of material removed at surgery. The tissues show
marked thickening with collagen proliferation, chronic inflammatory cell
infiltration and fibrin deposition (Quiles et al. 1978).

It is now appreciated that secondary inflammation and fibrosis occur
in lesser back pain problems, particularly in spinal stenosis when the
problem of bony narrowing of the nerve root canal may be exacerbated by
the thickening of the nerve root sheath (Epstein et al. 1978).
Similarly in lumbar spondylosis this secondary inflammatory change and
fibrosis may be so important that it has been suggested that the
recognised spectrum of arachnoiditis probably only represents the "tip
of the iceberg" of this common problem (Hoffman 1983).

## The fibrinolytic system and fibrin deposition

When tissues are damaged fibrinogen polymerises to form fibrin which is laid down in tissues. The fibrinolytic system is a complex cascade of reactions reponsible for the clearing of fibrin. In acute injury fibrin deposition is associated with a transient defect in the fibrinolytic system (Innes and Sevitt 1964). Usually within a few days or a couple of weeks after injury the fibrin is cleared and the secondary inflammation resolves.

Fibrin deposition is a common feature in chronic inflammation and it may have a possible pathogenic role. In particular it has been shown that in sensitised animals, intra-articular injection of both autologous and heterologous fibrin produced chronic arthritis (Dumonde and Glynn 1962). Persistence of fibrin in vessel walls and tissues may lead to impairment of diffusion of oxygen into the tissues and tissue anoxia (Browse 1983). The failure to clear fibrin in the normal way, therefore, could lead to chronicity of inflammation in damaged tissues.

## Fibrin studies in chronic back pain problems

Histological studies of specimens of nerve root sheaths removed at laminectomy has shown the presence of scar tissue with chronic inflammatory cell infiltration. However, in many of our specimens, we have found extensive deposits of fibrin intimately blending with the chronic inflammatory tissue. The appearance is very similar to that seen in venous lipodermatosclerosis, systemic sclerosis and other disorders. These observations have led us to study the fibrinolytic system in patients with severe chronic back pain syndromes.

Patients were studied in the morning, fasting, and not having eaten or smoked since the previous midnight. Blood was taken in a standard fashion and examined for parameters of fibrinolytic activity. In patients with chronic mechanical problems we found very marked evidence of a fibrinolytic defect (Jayson et al. 1984). In particular there was prolongation of the euglobulin clot lysis time and reduction of the fibrin plate lysis area. This could be responsible for the persistence of fibrin deposits in tissues and the chronicity of inflammation and fibrosis in involved areas.

The cause of this fibrinolytic defect is uncertain. It is possible that it preceded the development of the back problem and its presence led to the failure to clear fibrin, the chronicity of inflammation, and pain.   Alternatively, the defect may have developed in response to the injury, but persisted because the original insult remained; or was secondary to the inflammation itself or to other unknown factors. In this regard the association of back pain with smoking is of interest (Frymoyer 1983).   Smoking is associated with the development of a defect in the fibrinolytic system (Meade et al 1979); this may explain why smokers are more at risk of chronic back problems.

Analogies with other diseases

There are other conditions in which a similar pathogenic process appears important.   In particular in venous lipodermatosclerosis, in which there is chronic inflammation and fibrosis of the calf following a deep venous thrombosis, fibrin deposits may be demonstrated in the tissues and a similar fibrinolytic defect has been found (Browse 1983). Similar observations have been made in rheumatoid arthritis (Belch et al. 1986), systemic sclerosis (Jayson et al. 1985), and cutaneous vasculitis (Cunliffe et al. 1975). It, therefore, is possible that this is a mechanism of chronicity of inflammation which may occur in many different sites in the body.

FIBRINOLYTIC ENHANCEMENT THERAPY

The possible role of a fibrinolytic defect in these various conditions has led to trials of stimulation of the fibrinolytic system.   The drug Stanozolol has been used in venous lipodermatosclerosis, systemic sclerosis, rheumatoid arthritis and cutaneous vasculitis. In particular, in venous lipodermatosclerosis it has been shown to produce significant improvement in the fibrinolytic parameters in the blood, reduction in the amount of fibrin in the damaged tissues in the calf and clinical improvement.   These observations have led to studies of this form of treatment in patients requiring mechanical back pain syndromes.

Preliminary observations have been undertaken using Stanozolol which is a non-virilising anabolic steroid.   Unfortunately, it has mild androgenic effects and these have been a problem in some younger female patients.   It also occasionally disturbed the liver function tests. In some patients there have been remarkable improvements associated with correction of the fibrinolytic defect.   Others have failed to respond.

In using this form of treatment it appears to be pre-requisite to demonstrate the fibrinolytic defect and to follow the changes during treatment.  Improvements often take several months to occur and without such careful observations it is difficult to know whether fibrinolytic enhancement therapy is indicated and whether any benefit can be anticipated.


## HYPOTHESIS OF CHRONIC BACK PAIN (Figure 1)


These observations have led us to suggest that the spine may be damaged in a wide variety of different ways.  These may include disc prolapse, spondylosis, myelography, surgery, etc.  The damage will produce localised inflammation associated with fibrin deposition and a fibrinolytic defect.  In the normal way this is a transient event. With correction of the fibrinolytic defect there is resorption of the fibrin and clearing of the inflammation with resolution of the pain.

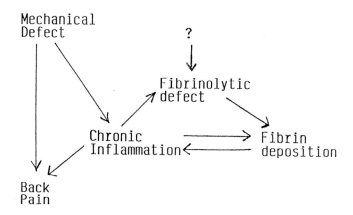

FIG. 1.  The inflammatory component of mechanical back problems.

However, in some patients the fibrinolytic defect persists.  This may be a consequence of the injury, the persistence of some noxious insult, the presence of chronic inflammation itself, treatment, smoking or some other unrecognised cause.  This is associated with failure to clear fibrin and persistent chronic inflammation and scar tissue which in turn will lead to chronic pain.

## CONCLUSIONS

It appears that secondary chronic inflammation is a common problem in patients with chronic mechanical back pain. This seems well established and it is possible that the fibrinolytic defect may be the mechanism or one of the mechanisms underlying its persistence. If this is correct, treatment aimed at correcting the fibrinolytic defect may offer a useful approach in the management of such patients.

## REFERENCES

Belch, J. J. F., Madhock, R., McArdle, B., McLaughlin, K., Kluft, C., Forbes, C. D. and Sturrock, R. D. (1986). The effect of increasing fibrinolysis in patients with rheumatoid arthritis: a double blind study of Stanozolol. Quarterly Journal of Medicine, 58: 19-27.

Bisla, R. S., Marchisello, P. J., Lockshin, M. D., Hart, D. M., Marcus, R. E. and Granda, J. (1976). Auto-immunological basis of disc degeneration. Clinical Orthopaedics and Related Research, 121: 205-211.

Browse, N. L. (1983). Venous ulceration. British Medical Journal, 286: 1920-1922.

Burton, C. V. (1978). Lumbo-sacral arachnoiditis. Spine, 3: 24-30.

Cunliffe, W. J., Dodman, B., Roberts, B. E. and Tetts, E. N. (1975). Clinical and laboratory double-blind investigation of fibrinolytic therapy of cutaneous vasculitis. In: Progress in Chemical Fibrinolysis and Thrombolysis. (Eds. Davidson, J. F., Samama, M. M. and Desmoyers, P. C.), Raven Press, New York, pp. 325-332.

Diamant, B., Karlsson, J. and Nachemson, A. (1968). Correlation between lactate levels and pH in discs of patients with lumbar rhizopathies. Experientia, 24: 1195-1196.

Dumonde, D. C. and Glynn, L. E. (1962). The production of arthritis in rabbits by an immunological reaction to fibrin. British Journal of Experimental Pathology, 43: 373-383.

Epstein, J. A., Epstein, B. S., Lavine, L. S., Rosenthal, A. D., Decker, R. E. and Carras, R. (1978). Obliterative arachnoiditis complicating lumbar spinal stenosis. Journal of Neurosurgery, 48: 252-258.

Frymoyer, J. W., Pope, M. H., Clements, J. H., Wilder, D. G., MacPherson, B. and Ashikaga, T. (1983). Risk factors in low back pain: An epidemiological study. Journal of Bone and Joint Surgery, 65-A: 213-218.

Goldie, I. (1958). Granulation tissue in the ruptured intervertebral disc. Acta Pathologica Scandinavica, 42: 302-304.

Hirsch, C. (1959). Studies on the pathology of low back pain. Journal of Bone and Joint Surgery, 41-B: 237-243.

Hoffman, G. S. (1983). Spinal arachnoiditis: What is the clinical spectrum? Spine, 8: 538-540.

Innes, D. and Sevitt, S. (1964). Coagulation and fibrinolysis in injured patients. Journal of Clinical Pathology, 17: 1-13.

Jayson, M. I. V., Keegan, A., Million, R. and Tomlinson, I. (1984). A fibrinolytic defect in chronic back pain syndromes. Lancet, ii: 1186-1187.

Jayson, M. I. V., Keegan, A. L., Holland, C. D., Longstaff, J., Taylor, L. and Gush, R. (1985). A study of Stanozolol therapy for systemic sclerosis and Raynaud's phenomenon. In: Progress in Fibrinolysis VII. (Eds. Davidson, J. F. et al.), Churchill Livingstone, Edinburgh, pp. 111-112.

Lawrence, J. S. (1977). Disc Disorders. In: Rheumatism in Populations. Heinemann, London. pp. 68-97.

Lindahl, O. (1966). Hyperalgesia of the lumbar nerve roots in sciatica.

Acta Orthopaedica Scandinavica, 37:   367–374.

Meade, T. W., Chakrabarti, R., Haines, A. P., North, W. R. S. and Stirling, Y. (1979).   Characteristics affecting fibrinolytic activity and plasma fibrinogen concentrations.   British Medical Journal, 1: 153–156.

Nachemson, A. (1969).   Intradiscal measurements of pH in patients with lumbar rhizopathies.   Acta Orthopaedica Scandinavica, 40:   23–42.

Quiles, M., Marchisello, P. J. and Tsairis, P. (1978).   Lumbar adhesive arachnoiditis.   Etiologic and pathologic aspects.   Spine, 3:   45–50.

## 36. LONG TERM RESULTS OF UNCEMENTED HIP REPLACEMENT

### P. A. Ring

### INTRODUCTION

Total replacement of the hip joint has been with us for 25 years, but no-one knows what the long term results are likely to be. Most of our older patients will die before their joints fail; few have the stamina of Sir Harry Platt, and most of the younger patients will outlive the surgeons performing the operation.

If uncemented hip replacement is to retain a place in orthopaedic surgery it must give a result which is comparable with that of the totally cemented joint. One cannot hope to better the results achieved by Sir John Charnley, but one should not do significantly worse. If by avoiding the use of bone cement there are advantages, this is a bonus.

Four thousand one hundred and forty-three uncemented hip replacements were inserted at the Unit in Dorking between 1964 and 1985. The mortality in hospital was 0·9%. Thirteen of these hips became infected, but there have been no deep-seated infections during the last 10 years. There were 6 post-operative dislocations, and 2 recurrent dislocations, and 1 patient sustained a partial sciatic palsy. The morbidity has clearly been low, and the relative simplicity of uncemented joint replacement and the speed with which the procedure can be performed may play some part in this. Of all these patients, 5·4% have come to revisional surgery, mainly for implant loosening.

### PREVIOUS IMPLANTS

The first of the implants inserted in 1964 was based on a Moore's prosthesis matched to a cup with a long, parallel screw thread inserted in the axial line of the pelvis. This cup was modified to give it a conical outer surface, and the axial screw became tapered to prevent fatigue. This principle of cup orientation and insertion has remained unchanged for more than 20 years. In 1966 the stem of the femoral component was narrowed, but at this time the implants, like those of McKee, were simply lapped together, and the frictional co-efficient was high. The results in these patients, 11 to 15 years later are seen in Table 1; 36% remained excellent, but 33% were poor.

Table 1

Prototype and Early Models

11-15 Year Review

|                            | Number | %  |
|----------------------------|--------|----|
| Excellent                  | 57     | 36 |
| Good                       | 37     | 23 |
| Fair                       | 13     | 8  |
| Poor, including revisions  | 53     | 33 |
| Lost to Review             | 25     |    |

The development of the apical bearing marked an important step forward in metal on metal joints; not only was the friction markedly lower, but the implants were interchangeable. A valgus configuration was also introduced on the femoral component, and 2 sizes of femoral stem became available. The results in this group of patients, reviewed from 7 to 10 years post-operatively were markedly better, and 87% of them can be regarded as acceptable (Table 2) although in only 67% was the full potential of a total hip replacement achieved.

The valgus configuration had two disadvantages; it increased the overall joint loading, and in some patients it produced a secondary valgus at the knee. It was replaced in 1969 by an implant with a conventional 135° neck-shaft angle, which was produced in 3 sizes, the acetabular component remaining unchanged. At 5 years (Table 3) 81% of these implants gave excellent results, they were comparable (Ring 1973) with the results of the cemented metal on metal articulation used by McKee (McKee and Chen 1973), but were certainly inferior to the results reported by Charnley (1979). At 10 years the proportion of excellent

Table 2

Valgus Configuration

7-10 Year Review

|  | Number | % |
|---|---|---|
| Excellent | 288 | 67 |
| Good | 85 | 20 |
| Fair | 26 | 6 |
| Poor, including revisions | 33 | 7 |
| Lost to Review | 31 | |

Table 3

Straight-Stem Series

5 Year Review

|  | Number | % |
|---|---|---|
| Excellent | 280 | 81 |
| Good | 50 | 14 |
| Fair | 10 | 3 |
| Poor, including revisions | 6 | 2 |
| Lost to Review | 14 | |

results had dropped to 67%, although 89% of the patients reviewed could be assessed as having acceptable function (Table 4). The radiographs at this point indicated that the majority of the acetabular components showed no change (Table 5) but on the femoral side almost 50% showed changes (Table 6), some of which were progressive.

The overall results of these implants remained inferior to those of the low friction arthroplasty, and in 1978, a series of 200 totally cemented metal on plastic implants were inserted in parallel with a similar number of uncemented joints. Each group has been assessed annually for 7 years. The initial results appeared comparable in these groups in terms of pain, motion and function, and the uncemented articulation, therefore, has been used in all primary replacements since that time.

Table 4

Straight-Stem Series

10 Year Review

|                          | Number | %  |
|--------------------------|--------|----|
| Excellent                | 248    | 67 |
| Good                     | 82     | 22 |
| Fair                     | 34     | 9  |
| Poor, including revisions| 8      | 2  |
| Lost to Review           | 34     |    |

Table 5

Metal on Metal Joints

Acetabular Changes - 10 Years

|                      | Number | %  |
|----------------------|--------|----|
| None                 | 349    | 93 |
| Upward displacement  | 10     | 3  |
| Medial displacement  | 6      | 2  |
| Loosening            | 7      | 2  |

Table 6

Metal on Metal Joints

Femoral Changes - 10 Years

|                    | Number | %  |
|--------------------|--------|----|
| None               | 207    | 55 |
| Sinking            | 76     | 20 |
| Calcar Pivot       | 66     | 18 |
| Calcar Resorption  | 62     | 17 |
| Loose              | 12     | 3  |

Some show 2 or more changes

## METAL ON PLASTIC JOINTS

The uncemented articulation is a 32 mm. implant.    The polyethylene acetabular component has external diameters of 45, 50, 55, and 60 mm., and retains the conical configuration but the mouth is offset.    The implant relies for primary fixation on the Freeman osseous peg.    The femoral component is available in 3 sizes, and has no fenestrations (Ring 1983).    The operative technique is similar to that employed for the metal on metal articulation, and the fate of the 1488 hip arthroplasties inserted between 1979 and 1985 is indicated in Table 7.

### Table 7

UPM Hips

1979-1985

|                     | Number | %  |
|---------------------|--------|----|
| Died in Hospital    | 13     | 1  |
| Lost to Review      | 45     | 3  |
| Awaiting assessment | 50     | 3  |
| Reviewed            | 1380   | 93 |
|                     |        |    |
| Total               | 1488   |    |

The results in the 1380 patients reviewed 1 to 7 years post-operatively (Table 8), indicated that 93% of these hips were functioning normally, with a 0·5% annual revision rate.    Clinically these hips were superior to the metal on metal articulations.

Polyethylene bearing directly on bone appeared to be acceptable, and during the first post-operative year a dense band of bone developed to support the acetabular component.    There was a favourable response in the presence of an acetabular protrusion, and if the cup was located to restore the normal axis of joint movement bone developed medially, and the protrusion resolved.    Even in the presence of gross acetabular destruction reconstitution occurred without grafting, and the response of the cancellous bone to uncemented implantation, in general, was favourable (Sharp et al. 1984), and the need to graft was rare.

There have been 5 acetabular failures (Table 9), 2 from poor operative technique, and 3 in which the implants loosened without obvious cause.   In each of the latter erosion occurred, and although  2 were successfully revised with cups with oversized pegs, the third eventually had to be converted into a pseudarthrosis.   Bone erosion in uncemented acetabular components was rare, and was confined to thin-walled cups with a small external diameter, but there appeared to be some advantage with small implants, in shielding the plastic from bone.

## Table 8

UPM Hips

1979-1985

1-7 Year Review

|           | Number | %    |
|-----------|--------|------|
| Excellent | 1286   | 93   |
| Good      | 65     | 5    |
| Fair      | 9      | 0·5  |
| Revised   | 20     | 1·5  |

## Table 9

UPM Hips

Acetabular Failures

| Cause              | Treatment    | Result       |
|--------------------|--------------|--------------|
| Poor Coning        | Reconed      | Satisfactory |
| Inadequate Support | Grafted      | Satisfactory |
| Peg Fracture       | Oversize Peg | Satisfactory |
| Erosions           | Oversize Peg | Satisfactory |
| Erosions           | Oversize Peg | Failed       |

Femoral failures have been greater in number and have all been due to loosening.   Of the 18 femoral components requiring revisional  surgery, 5 have been due to technical failures at the time of primary surgery. Revisional surgery was technically easy (Jones 1981),  and  in  general

successful (Table 10).    Cement was used in the older patients,  and  in
the  younger  an  implant  with mesh in the trochanteric region, with or
without grafting.

### Table 10

### UPM Hips

Revisional Surgery

| Mode | Result |
|---|---|
| Femoral Cemented | Excellent 14 |
| Died       1 | |
| Femoral Uncemented | Excellent  2 |
| Good       1 | |
| Acetabular Uncemented | Excellent  4 |
| Failed   1 | |
| 3 Revisions of both components | |

### CONCLUSIONS

The use of an uncemented implant during the last 20  years  appeared  to
have 3 advantages:

(i)    The morbidity was small.

(ii)   The acetabulum responded favourably to a prosthesis which was
       sound on insertion, and relocated the centre of joint movement
       back to the anatomical position.

(iii)  Revisional surgery was easy, and on the whole successful, but
       in the elderly the femoral side may demand the use of cement.

Failures  of  a  metallic  acetabular component were rare, and in the
long term were confined to asymptomatic migration without erosion.    If
polyethylene fails, it will fragment and produce erosions, and there may
be some merit in shielding polyethylene from bone.

The femoral side of the articulation presented greater  problems  and
in  some  patients  press-fit  implants  failed.    Some form of osseous
entrapment or ingrowth system confined to the  trochanteric  region  may
diminish this risk.

Although the primary results of metal on metal joints were clinically inferior to the current metal on plastic, failures in these patients, when they occurred, presented in the first few post-operative years, and late failure requiring revisional surgery was exceptionally rare. With more than 1000 of these patients still on annual review, most with implants inserted between 10 and 20 years ago, fewer than one per annum come to any exchange procedure. The quality of the articular surface in these joints did not change with the passage of time, and debris formation was minimal. They may still have a place in the management of the patient with an expectation of life of 40 or 50 years, although in the older patient, the merits of metal on plastic, whether cemented or not, outweigh most of the risks associated with late erosion of bone.

## REFERENCES

Charnley, J. (1979). Low friction arthroplasty of the hip. Springer-Verlag, Berlin, Heidelberg, New York.

Jones, J. M. (1981). Revisional total hip replacement for failed Ring arthroplasty. Journal of Bone and Joint Surgery, 61-A: 1029-1034.

McKee, G. K. and Chen, S. C. (1973). The statistics of the McKee-Farrar method of total hip replacement. Clinical Orthopaedics and Related Research, 95: 26-33.

Ring, P. A. (1973). Total replacement of the hip joint. Clinical Orthopaedics and Related Research, 95: 34-37.

Ring, P. A. (1983). Ring U.P.M. total hip arthroplasty. Clinical Orthopaedics and Related Research, 176: 115-123.

Sharp, D. J., Porter, K. M. and Duke, R. F. N. (1984). The resolution of protrusio acetabuli treated with Ring's hip prosthesis. Journal of Bone and Joint Surgery, 66-B: 635-638.

## 37.CHEVRON OSTEOTOMY OF THE GREATER TROCHANTER

I. S. Fyfe
M. R. K. Karpinski
G. Newton

## INTRODUCTION

Trochanteric osteotomy for approach to the hip joint in total hip arthroplasty facilitates exposure in certain difficult clinical situations such as revisional arthroplasty, hip dysplasia and protrusio acetabuli, providing better access to both proximal femur and acetabulum. Osteotomy also allows adjustment of trochanteric position, adjustment of abductor tension, easier correction of rotational deformity and better prosthetic alignment with a lesser risk of dislocation. Posterior approaches to the hip can be associated with dislocation rates as high as 7·5% (Robinson et al. 1980).

A direct comparison of osteotomised and non-osteotomised patients showed an increased abductor efficiency following successful re-attachment of the trochanter (Mallory 1974). Osteotomy, however, increased the operating time, blood loss and length of hospital stay (Parker et al. 1976, Wiesman et al. 1978) and was associated with an incidence of non-union or detachment. Amstutz and Maki (1978) reported a significant reduction of abductor power in 50% of non-unions. Ritter and colleagues (1981) found improved gait with successful re-attachments but little difference in pain, range of movements or activity levels. Non-union incidences as high as 9·7% have been documented and are usually associated with failure of fixation devices. Considerable ingenuity has been applied to the design of re-attachment techniques in an attempt to reduce the rotational forces acting across the osteotomy site. Single wire techniques (Coventry), vertical horizontal locking two-wire techniques (Amstutz) and triple wire techniques (Harris) have all been described. The Charnley wire technique itself has progressed from a single to a triple wire method.

The efficiency of four such techniques tested by Markolf and co-authors (1979) suggested that the more complex triple wiring was more resistant to pull off.

Sir John Charnley recognised that the trochanter was subjected to a rotational shearing stress as a result of muscle pull and hip movement, especially in flexion, and advocated the use of a trochanteric bolt system to reduce this effect. Other devices such as the Votz bolt and Getschner plate have been developed. Modification of the osteotomy itself is another approach to this problem. Debeyre and Doliveux (1954) suggested a V-osteotomy which was subsequently renamed the "dihedral self-stabilising osteotomy" by Weber and Stühmer (1979), and the "bi-planar intracapsular osteotomy" by Wroblewski. The V-osteotomy produced inherent stability to shearing stress but could produce a rather delicate shell of bone easily damaged by fixation.

"The best hope for the future would seem to be in designing the osteotomy to possess an inherent stability against forces tending to produce displacement and combining this with improved methods of fixation" (Hamblen 1984).

The Dall Miles cable grip system (Dall and Miles 1983) is such a strong fixation technique, but our experience combining this powerful device with a standard osteotomy was a little disappointing. Of the first 100 re-attachements using the grip, 25 failed: 8 from technical error, 4 following dislocation and 13 from fixation failure presumably due to cyclical loading with shearing stress.

## TECHNIQUE

The Chevron, or inverted V, osteotomy (Figures 1 and 2) was designed to produce inherent stability to resist shearing stresses and yet to produce a fragment of trochanter sufficiently strong to enable use of the cable grip system and other devices to best effect. The technique also leaves the majority of the posterior soft tissues intact giving added stability to the arthroplasty.

Through a direct lateral approach, the fascia lata is split in line with the skin incision and retracted to expose the vastus lateralis ridge which is defined with electro-cautery. The interval between the gluteus medius and the other soft tissues is opened, the trochanteric

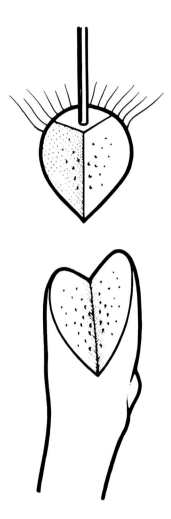

FIG. 1.  The Chevron osteotomy.

fossa defined and a Steinmann pin advanced from the mid-point of the
vastus lateralis ridge laterally to the trochanteric fossa (Figure 3).
The Chevron osteotomy with its apex medially placed is then performed
using either an oscillating or a reciprocating saw.   An anterior and
posterior cut is made preferably passing medial to the pin thus leaving
the anterior and posterior lips of the greater trochanter in situ
(Figure 2).    The trochanteric fragment can then be elevated using the
Steinmann pin as a retractor, exposing the deep 'V' in the lateral
surface of the trochanteric bed (Figure 1).    The capsule is then opened
fully and resected as necessary.

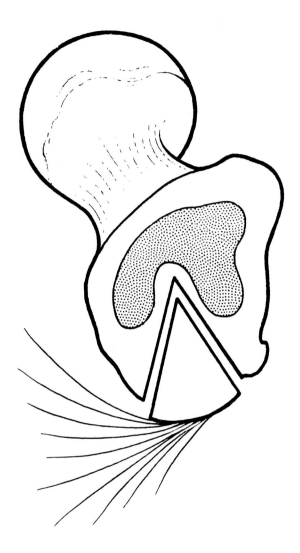

FIG. 2.   View of Chevron osteotomy from above.

On completion of the arthroplasty, the trochanteric fragment  may  be
brought  down  using  the  Steinmann  pin  allowing  adjustment  of  the
trochanteric position with ease within  the  grooved  trochanteric  bed.
The  trochanter should be re-attached using a strong fixation technique.
If a Dall-Miles cable grip is used the grip must be bedded well into the
trochanteric  fragment  and  the  cables  cut  as  short  as  possible if
bursitis is not to occur.

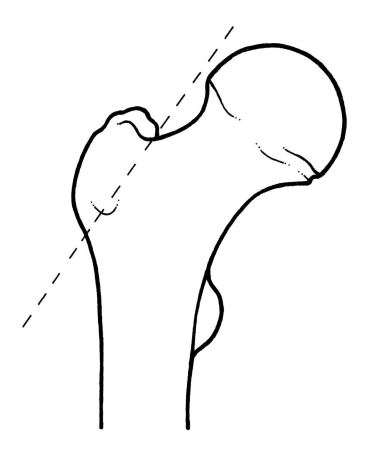

FIG. 3.    The line of osteotomy.


## RESULTS

Chevron osteotomies were performed on 100 consecutive patients at two centres by the authors.   The Dall–Miles trochanter cable grip system was used for re-attachment.   The patients were reviewed at a minimum of six months following surgery.   The majority of arthroplasties were primary procedures, only 12 being revisional procedures in which the greater trochanter had not been previously removed.   The most common underlying pathology was osteoarthritis.   Sixty-two patients were female with an average age of 71 years; 38 were male with an average age of 60 years.   The average weight of the men was higher (75·2Kgs) when compared with the females, but this did not take into account their somato-typing.     Elderly   and   overweight   females   predominated.    Hip radiographs were procured at two, four and six months following surgery. Continuity   of   trabecula   was   accepted   as   evidence   of   bony   union. Trochanteric separation of 3 cms was regarded as non-union;    separation of less than 3 cms as fibrous union.

Difficult   clinical situations presented themselves for rectification including revision of a loose prosthesis with considerable bone loss   in an   elderly   lady,   and   a loose prosthesis in a young patient following congenital dislocation of the hip with poor bone stock.    Ideal fixation resulted in bony union with an excellent pain-free range of movement.

Non-union   occurred in 5 patients;   2 following falls, 2 attributable to technical errors, and 1 due to a   dramatic   wire   failure.    Fibrous union was seen in 3 asymptomatic patients.   Wire breakage occurred in 4 other situations but produced no   problems.    Significant   trochanteric bursitis was found in 2 patients and was attributable to poor cable grip seating or inadequate trimming   of   the   wires.    Minimal   trochanteric bursitis   was experienced by 12 other patients.    The 2 technical errors were multiple saw cuts within the soft   bone   of   a   rheumatoid   patient producing   fragmentation   of   the   fragment   and a loose proximal cable. The 1 catastrophic wire failure was only explicable   in   terms   of   wire fatigue.


## CONCLUSIONS

The   Chevron   osteotomy   described combined with a Dall-Miles trochanter cable grip produced satisfactory trochanteric re-attachment   in   95%   of patients   and is presented as a useful technique in the armamentarium of the hip arthroplasty surgeon.


## REFERENCES

Amstutz, H. C. and   Maki,   S.   (1978).   Complications   of   trochanteric osteotomy   in total hip replacement.   Journal of Bone and Joint Surgery, 60-A:   214-216.

Dall, D. M. and Miles, A. W. (1983). Re-attachment of the greater trochanter:  the use of the trochanter cable grip system. Journal of Bone and Joint Surgery, 65-B:  55-59.

Debeyre, J. and Doliveux, P. (1954). Les arthroplasties de la hanche: étude critique à propos de 200 cas opérés. Editions Medical Flammarion, Paris.

Hamblen, D. L. (1984). In: Complications of total hip replacement. (Ed. Ling, R. S. M.). Churchill Livingstone, Edinburgh, pp. 91-99.

Mallory, T. H. (1974). Total hip replacement with and without trochanteric osteotomy. Clinical Orthopaedics and Related Research, 103:  133-135.

Markolf, K. L., Hirschowitz, D. L. and Amstutz, H. C. (1979). Mechanical stability of the greater trochanter following osteotomy and re-attachment with wiring. Clinical Orthopaedics and Related Research, 141:  111-121.

Parker, H. G., Wiesman, H. G., Ewald, F. C., Thomas, W. H. and Sledge, C. B. (1976). Comparison of pre-operative, intra-operative and early post-operative total hip replacements with and without trochanteric osteotomy. Clinical Orthopaedics and Related Research, 121:  44-49.

Ritter, M. A., Gioe, T. J. and Stringer, E. A. (1981). Functional significance of non-union of the greater trochanter. Clinical Orthopaedics and Related Research, 159:  177-182.

Robinson, R. P., Robinson, H. J. and Salvati, E. A. (1980). Comparison of the trans-trochanteric and posterior approaches for total hip replacement. Clinical Orthopaedics and Related Research, 147:  143-147.

Weber, B. G. and Stühmer, G. (1979). Improvements in total hip prosthesis implantation technique. A cement-proof seal for the lower medullary cavity and a dihedral self-stabilising trochanteric osteotomy. Archives of Orthopaedic and Traumatic Surgery, 93:  185-189.

Wiesman, H. J., Simon, S. R., Ewald, F. C., Thomas, W. H. and Sledge, C. B. (1978). Total hip replacement with and without osteotomy of the greater trochanter. Clinical and biomechanical comparison in the same patients. Journal of Bone and Joint Surgery, 60-A: 203-210.

## 38. FROM PRIMARY TO REVISION SURGERY

B. M. Wroblewski
P. Shelley

## INTRODUCTION

November 1985 saw 23 year results of the Charnley low friction arthroplasty (LFA). Since the introduction of the method into clinical practice numerous advances have been made to improve the long term results. The recent upsurge of uncemented total hip arthroplasties reflects designers' attempts to move away from the use of cement for component fixation. Although some of them are due to the genuine desire to establish alternative methods, others probably stem from lack of understanding of the properties of the acrylic cement and the role it plays in component fixation. There can be little doubt that the report, which has shown that at least 25% of the sockets of the Charnley LFA will eventually fail, because of loosening, has also contributed to this change (Charnley 1975).

In order that any new method can be meaningfully assessed it is essential to understand the evolution, the results and the complications of the Charnley LFA, the hip replacement which has the longest follow-up record. To date over 20,000 operations have been carried out in the Centre for Hip Surgery. This article reviews the long term results, complications, lessons learned and outlines the prospects for the future. This knowledge will allow other methods to be assessed meaningfully. Without it, the surgeon and the patient alike, may be subjected to unnecessary experiences and without any guarantee of long term success.

In the design of Charnley LFA the low frictional torque principle was the main theme, while in the surgical technique reconstruction of the mechanics of the hip joint was of utmost importance. Both aimed, ultimately, at avoiding loosening of components. The immediate clinical success established this procedure as a method of choice in the treatment of a destroyed arthritic hip joint.


## CLINICAL RESULTS

A review of 116 Charnley LFA's in 93 patients with an average follow-up of 16·6 years (range 15-21 years) has shown that pain relief was complete in 83·6% while 11% had not more than occasional discomfort. The remaining 5·4% were considered to have failed and probably in need of revision in the future (Wroblewski 1986). Considering that these cases represented results from early stages of the development of the technique, there is reason for optimism. Radiographic appearances on the acetabular side left no room for complacency - 21·6% of sockets were considered to be loose as judged by serial radiographs. The reason for this has become obvious when wear of the socket was studied in some detail.


### Dislocation

This complication, so often levelled at the 22·25 mm. head diameter of the design, had not presented as a serious problem.

In a review of 14,672 Charnley LFA's (Fraser and Wroblewski 1981) the incidence of post-operative dislocation was 0.63% (92 cases) and only 16 (0·11%) required re-operation. (It must be stressed, however, that a number of them dislocated at least once more following revision.) The majority of dislocations came to revision within the first three post-operative years although a handful occurred very much later (Figure 1). The number of revisions for dislocation is on the increase in line with the increasing number of revisions, from all sources, being carried out.

Revision for recurrent dislocation remains one of the most taxing procedures, demanding attention to detail at every stage, and often a full scale revision.


### Infection

This is a reflection of various aspects of patient selection, environment and possibly of the surgical technique, as well as various prophylactic methods being used. As such it is not an integral part

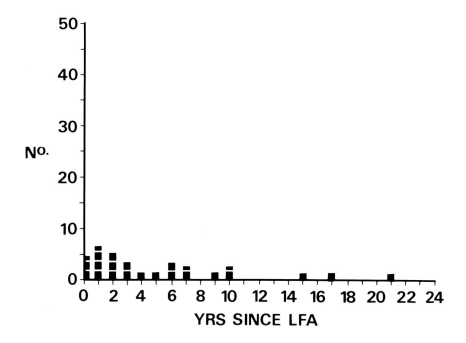

FIG. 1.    Revisions for dislocation.
           Incidence in relation to post-operative follow-up.

of the long term results of the method although an inseparable  part  of
the principles laid down by the late Professor Sir John Charnley.

Fracture of the stem

The  incidence was 1·6% in the group of patients with a follow-up longer
than 11 years.   The mechanism of the fracture (Wroblewski  1979a),  the
method  of  management  (Wroblewski  1979b) and various clinical aspects
have been reviewed (Charnley 1975, Wroblewski 1982).

    This complication was extremely  rare  in  the  first  post-operative
year.   It  peaked  in the eighth post-operative year and in almost all
the patients with normal  function  it  no  longer  appeared  after  the
eleventh year (Figure 2).

    This pattern of incidence of stem fracture suggests a "fatigue limit"
phenomenon, indicating that the stainless steel component  was  stressed
in  a  non-corrosive environment.   If this is the case, there is little
indication for the  use  of  apparently  stronger,  and  certainly  more
expensive metals.

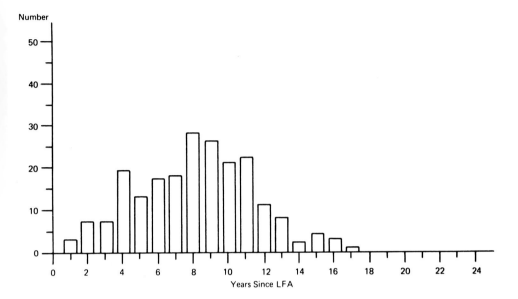

FIG. 2.    Revisions for fractured stems.
           Incidence in relation to the post-operative follow-up.

What is more interesting, is this complication as part of the evolution of the Charnley LFA. The first case presented in 1968, 6 years and some 2,500 cases after introduction of the method into clinical practice (Figure 3). From the ninth to the nineteenth year (1971-1981) its incidence steadily increased and then fell dramatically over the next 4 years.

Introduction of the cold-formed high nitrogen content stainless steel (ORTRON - Chas. F. Thackray Limited) for the stem manufacture, flanged stem design, and improvement in the method of stem fixation (Wroblewski and Van der Rijt 1984) are only now becoming apparent. There have been no fractures of the ORTRON prosthesis.

Loosening of the stem

This has been regarded as the most common complication in many series. It is not so with the Charnley design and technique. To date fewer than 90 are known to have been revised for aseptic loosening. None have come to revision in the first post-operative year, the first stem being changed in 1968, the sixth year of the technique (Figure 4).

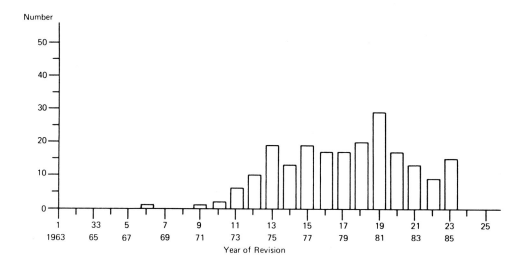

FIG. 3.    Revisions for fracture stems over 23 years of the Charnley LFA technique.    The top row of figures on the "X" axis represents the number of years since the Charnley LFA was first introduced.

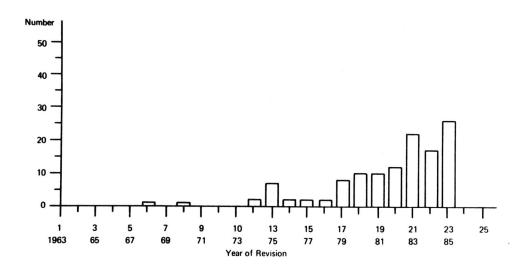

FIG. 4.    Revisions for loose stems over 23 years of the Charnley LFA technique.

The  incidence has gradually increased up to 1985, the twenty third year
of the operation.   The results due to the improvements  in  the  design
(flanged  stem) and the stem fixation (Wroblewski and Van der Rijt 1984)
are not yet coming through in  clinical  results  (Figure  5).    (There
always  is  a  time  lag between a new method and its effect on the long
term results.)

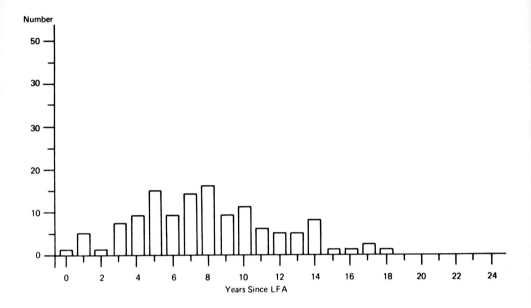

FIG. 5.    Revisions for loose stems.
           Incidence in relation to the post-operative follow-up.

Loosening of the socket
This probably more than any other complication has been the major factor
that  has  stirred  surgeons  to  seek  a cementless arthroplasty.   The
incidence peaks in the eighth post-operative year and gradually declines
with  the  increasing  follow-up  (Figure  6).    As with the mechanical
complications it first became an indication for revision in 1968  -  six
years  and  some 2,500 cases after the introduction of the Charnley LFA.
Its incidence is on the increase.

    High density polyethylene, introduced after rapidly  wearing  Teflon,
became  the material of choice for the socket, and although wear studies
have been carried out there was little to suggest that this  was  likely
to become one of the main long term problems.

    The reasons for the increasing incidence of socket loosening has been

presented elsewhere (Wroblewski 1985a) and are related to socket wear.
As the metal head bores for itself a roughly cylindrical path in the
plastic socket, the angular range of movements becomes gradually
restricted.    The neck of the stem impinges on the socket rim, and the
shock loading and levering loosens the socket at the bone–cement
junction.    The correlation between the depth of socket wear and the
incidence of socket migration has already been pointed out (Wroblewski
1985a and 1985b), and supports the observation.    Damage of the head of
the femoral component is a potent cause of wear.

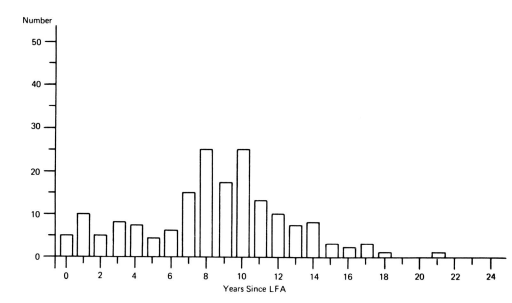

FIG. 6.    Revisions for loose sockets.
           Incidence in relation to the post-operative follow-up.

## WHAT ARE THE PROSPECTS FOR THE FUTURE?

There is little doubt that if the incidence of loosening of the
components is to be reduced their fixation at the primary operation must
be improved.    To this end flanged stem design, intramedullary bone
block and the Ogee-flanged socket are of clear benefit.
      Introduction of high nitrogen content stainless steel and cold
forming process for the manufacture of the stem (Ortron - Chas. F.
Thackray Limited) has allowed reduction of the diameter of the neck of

the stem from 12·5 to 10 mm. which in practical terms amounts to 3 mm. extra of plastic wear and 15 years on the "life" of the socket (Wroblewski 1985).

The obvious next step in the evolution of the Charnley LFA is to search for materials in order to reduce friction and wear still further. Surgeons undertaking other procedures or attempting to investigate alternative methods of component fixation must bear in mind that 6 years clinical experience and some 2,500 cases without revision for mechanical reasons, is the minimum required to emulate the results of the earliest method of the Charnley LFA. Frequent changes of design and short follow-up of small series do not inspire confidence.

## REFERENCES

Charnley, J. (1975). Fracture of femoral prostheses in total hip replacement. A clinical study. Clinical Orthopaedics and Related Research, 111: 105-120.

Charnley, J. (1978). Low friction arthroplasty of the hip. Theory and practice. Springer Verlag, Berlin, pp. 41-90.

Fraser, G. and Wroblewski, B. M. (1981). Revision of the Charnley low friction arthroplasty for recurrent or irreducible dislocation. Journal of Bone and Joint Surgery, 63-B: 552-555.

Wroblewski, B. M. (1979a). The mechanism of fracture of the femoral prosthesis in total hip replacement. International Orthopaedics, 3: 137-139.

Wroblewski, B. M. (1979b). A method of management of the fracture stem in total hip replacement. Clinical Orthopaedics and Related Research, 141: 71-73.

Wroblewski, B. M. (1982). Fractured stem in total hip replacement. A clinical review of 120 cases. Acta Orthopaedica Scandinavica, 53: 279-284.

Wroblewski, B. M. (1985a). Direction and rate of socket wear in Charnley low friction arthroplasty. Journal of Bone and Joint Surgery, 67-B: 757-761.

Wroblewski, B. M. (1985b). Charnley low friction arthroplasty in the young patient with degenerative hip disease. (Eds. Sevastik & Goldie). Almqvist and Wiksell International, Stockholm, Sweden.

Wroblewski, B. M. (1986). Fifteen to twenty one year results of the Charnley low friction arthroplasty. Clinical Orthopaedics and Related Research, 211: 30-35.

Wroblewski, B. M. and Van der Rijt, A. (1984). Intramedullary cancellous bone block to improve femoral stem fixation in Charnley low friction arthroplasty. Journal of Bone and Joint Surgery, 66-B: 639-644.

## 39. WEAR AS A CAUSE OF FAILURE IN TOTAL HIP ARTHROPLASTY

P. D. Wilson, Jr.
C. M. Rimnac
T. M. Wright

## INTRODUCTION

Wear of the polyethylene acetabular component of a total hip arthroplasty has received little attention, and, in fact, has classically been dismissed as an insignificant clinical problem (Charnley 1979, Cupic 1979). Radiographic measurements of wear in several long-term studies of Charnley total hip replacements have concluded that the average wear rate is low, typically from 0·1 to 0·2 mm. per annum, though in each series a small percentage of the components wore at three or four times this average rate (Charnley and Halley 1975, Cupic 1979, Salvati et al. 1981).

An experimental report on the radiographic measure of wear reported wide variations, suggesting that such measurements were too imprecise to be valid (Clarke et al. 1976), but this observation was refuted by Wroblewski's study of the comparison of radiographic wear rates compared with direct measurements made on the retrieved components after revision surgery in 22 cases (Wroblewski 1985). In that study, the sockets removed after an average of 7 years in vivo, with a range from 3 to 11 years. He found a close correlation between the two measurements and determined a mean wear rate from the direct measurements of 0·19 mm. per annum, with a range of 0·017 mm. to 0·52 mm.. However, no cases were cited in which the cause of failure could be attributed to the wear process itself.

The mean total wear rate in Clarac and colleagues' (1986) tenfold radiographic magnification study of 123 Charnley total hip replacements after 10 to 12 years was 1·1 mm., but their report included at least 8 cases which exhibited wear of 3 mm. or more. They also reported no cases of failure due to wear.

In a 15 year follow-up of the first 100 Charnley total hip arthroplasties carried out at The Hospital for Special Surgery, McCoy and co-authors (unpublished data) found that 27 of 32 original sockets examined radiographically exhibited wear. The average wear for all sockets was 1·56 mm. (0 – 8·5 mm.). Excluding the 5 sockets which did not exhibit any wear, the average total wear was 1·85 mm. over 15 years.

Five cases of fracture of polyethylene sockets have been reported in the literature, but these have all dealt with 32 mm. bearing prostheses and Mueller type sockets (Collins et al. 1982, Muzafer 1985, Salvati et al. 1979, Stout and Marsh 1981). The senior author has removed one fractured Charnley type acetabular component, but this seemed secondary to loosening rather than to wear. Recently, one case of a fractured Charnley socket secondary to full thickness wear has been reported (Moreland and Jinnah 1986).

This paper describes 2 patients in whom excessive wear of the acetabular components of Charnley total hip prostheses led directly to failure, through granulomatous destruction of the roof and walls of the acetabulum, in one patient by secondary loosening and in the other by pain and limp without loosening.


## PATIENTS


### Case presentations

**Patient 1:** A 44 year old woman, average 75± 7 kgms. during 10 years follow-up and suffering from severe unremitting ankylosing spondylitis which required corticosteroids throughout her course, underwent a right total hip arthroplasty in 1973, using a cobalt alloy femoral component and a polyethylene acetabular component. She did well clinically, but by $2\frac{1}{2}$ years a thin bone-cement radiolucency was noted in Zone I. Radiographs taken at 6 years showed a small iliac granuloma and slight wear of the socket, but she was asymptomatic and walked without a limp. By 8 years, the granuloma had progressed and the superior marker wire of the socket had broken. By 9 years, the iliac roof had collapsed and the cup had dislodged and become painfully loose, requiring revision (Figure 1).

The contralateral hip had received a total hip arthroplasty 2 years previously. At the time of last radiographic evaluation (11 years

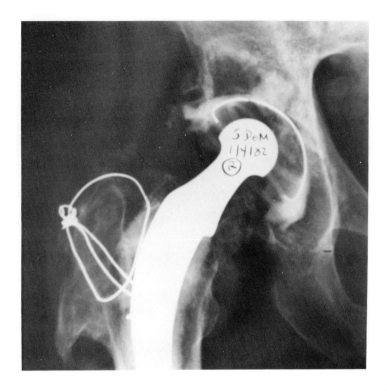

FIG. 1. Patient 1: Nine years post-operative. The iliac roof has collapsed. Note the proximal migration of socket, the wear of the socket and the fracture of the socket marker wire.

post-operatively), the left hip showed minimal socket wear and no evidence of granuloma. The patient died 9 months after her right revision total hip replacement of causes unrelated to her hip surgery.

Patient 2: A 63 year old, 64 kgm. active male physician with sequelae of treated congenital dislocated hip underwent one-stage bilateral Charnley low friction arthroplasties in 1972, using cobalt alloy femoral components and polyethylene acetabular components. Rather extensive subchondral fibromucoid cystic changes were noted in the left iliac roof pre- and post-operatively (Figure 2a). At 1 year, there was minimal demarcation of the left socket-bone cement interface, but no change in the appearance of the ilium. By $3\frac{1}{2}$ years there was minimal wear. Although there was no definite progression of the demarcation changes, a small granuloma was noted in the superolateral aspect of the left acetabulum. The patient had no symptoms and walked without a limp. At 7 years, progression of the wear and granuloma were noted, but there

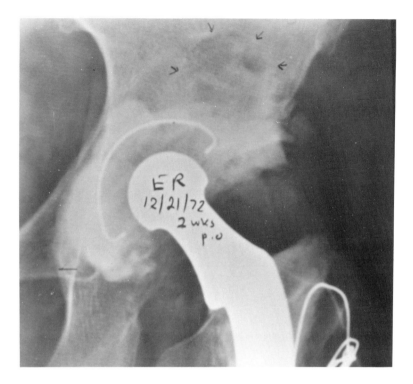

FIG. 2a. Patient 2: Two weeks post-operative. Note residua of osteoarthritic fibrocystic disease in ilium over acetabulum.

was no migration and only minimal progression of the demarcation. By 11 years, the granulomatous changes in the left ilium were much more striking, as was the amount of wear, but there was still no evidence of socket migration or tilting. The patient had retired from his practice and had moved to a rural area, where he carried on normal activities and was able to cover for 4 fellow physicians when they went on vacation. At $12\frac{1}{2}$ years, he had some left hip pain but felt that it was tolerable. His activity level was the same, but he now walked with a left-sided limp. There was severe destruction of the left iliac roof and of the acetabular walls (Figure 2b). Revision was recommended for fear that a catastrophe was imminent. At operation, the socket was found to be well-fixed in Zones II and III and had to be chiseled and burred out of the bone. There was extensive granulomatous destruction of acetabular bone, but a reconstruction was carried out using an acetabular screen and autogenous and allogenous bone grafts.

The opposite right hip was 14 years post-operative at last evaluation and was asymptomatic and fully functional. Radiographs showed no

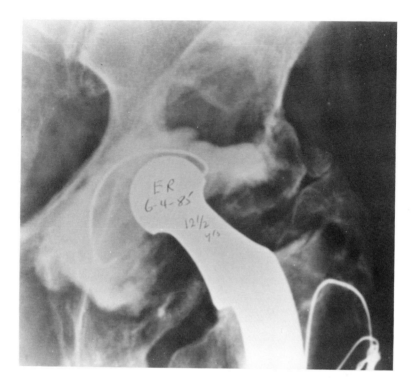

Fig. 2b.    Patient 2:  Twelve and one-half years post-operative.    Note
marked superolateral wear and  increased  size  of  granuloma.    Socket
remains well-fixed in Zones II and III.

significant loosening, socket migration or tilting, or femoral component
subsidence.    However, there was about 3 mm. of superior socket wear and
an  ischial granuloma of considerable proportions, which however had not
affected socket stability or innominate bone strength.

## Pathological findings

Pathological studies from both patients showed  extensive  granulomatous
tissue    containing    refractile    foreign    material    consistent with
polyethylene debris.    The pathological findings were  similar  in  both
cases,   except   that in the first the socket was grossly loose, while in
the second the   socket   was   still   rigidly   fixed to the medial   and
posterior   acetabular   walls   without an appreciable intervening fibrous
membrane.    Both granulomas were composed of   grumous   yellow,   somewhat
friable   soft tissue, adjacent to tough fibrous scar and bone fragments.
Microscopic study revealed necrotic tissue and granulation   tissue   with

focal histiocytic and giant cell responses to cement and refractile material identified as polyethylene on the basis of its morphological characteristics. Polyethylene debris dominated the sections in the second case, where socket loosening was not a factor and, therefore, cement abrasion was not as important a contributor of particulate debris.

Both polyethylene sockets were deeply worn in a superior direction with the wear having penetrated full thickness in the second patient, but not quite completely in the first. The bearing surfaces were severely burnished superiorly, while machining marks from manufacture of the sockets were still present in the inferior margins of the bearing surface.

Both sockets were directly measured at the point of maximum wear. The maximum change in cup thickness was 4·7 mm. for Patient 1 and 7·2 mm. for Patient 2, whereas the pre-revision anteroposterior radiographs (accounting for magnification) showed maximum changes in cup thickness of 3·8 mm. and 6·9 mm. respectively. The change in cup thickness was then measured in every available post-operative anteroposterior radiograph for each patient (7 follow-up radiographs for Patient 1 and 11 follow-up radiographs for Patient 2) to determine the average rate of wear per annum. In both cases, linear regression analysis of the resulting thickness versus time data gave a correlation coefficient of greater than 0·96. The average annual wear rate was found to be 0·42 mm. for Patient 1 and 0·53 mm. for Patient 2. These rates are several times greater than the average annual rate of wear reported by Wroblewski (1985) although they fall within the range of wear rates he reported.


## DISCUSSION

Extensive accumulation of polyethylene debris with consequent destructive osteolysis is worrying and has been previously reported elsewhere (Willert 1977, Wroblewski 1979, Remagen and Morscher 1984, Johanson et al. 1987). Wear debris accumulates in the surrounding tissue with time and the amount of debris is related to patient weight. In the 2 cases presented, radiographic measurements of wear showed a positive correlation with time from surgery. Similarly, in a study of

75 retrieved acetabular cups, positive correlations were found between the amount and severity of surface damage to the articulating surface and both time since implantation and patient weight (Wright et al. 1985). Several factors appear to affect the amount of debris generated from wear. These include the conformity between the articulating surfaces, the size of the bearing, the thickness of the polyethylene component and metal-backing (Bartel et al. 1982, 1986).

Physical factors may also affect the generation of debris. The molecular weight correlated with the wear resistance of polyethylene (Rose et al. 1980, Rose 1983).

The lack of excessive wear leading to failure in the contralateral hip arthroplasties in these 2 patients underscores the variability in the wear process. There are at least two possible explanations for the differences in wear. The original conformities between the bearings and sockets may have been significantly different. This would have affected the original stresses experienced by the polyethylene sockets and, therefore, the initial wear rate. However, as wear continued, the surfaces became conforming and the stress states should have been similar. Another explanation is that the original molecular weights were different. This difference could have affected both the wear rate and the rate of degradation.

Failure caused directly by polyethylene wear must be considered a rare complication, occurring mainly in total hip arthroplasties with 22·25 mm. bearings. Stress analysis suggested that a 28 mm. bearing would reduce the amount of wear and, therefore, the possibility of failure (Bartel et al. 1986). As total hip replacements survive for longer times, the incidence of this complication may increase.

## REFERENCES

Bartel, D. L., Wright, T. M. and Edwards, D. (1982). The effect of metal backing on stresses on polyethylene acetabular components. In: The Hip. Proceedings of the 11th Hip Society Open Meeting. C. V. Mosby Company, St. Louis, pp. 229-239.

Bartel, D. L., Bicknell, V. L. and Wright, T. M. (1986). The effect of conformity, thickness and material on stresses in ultra high molecular weight components for total joint replacement. Journal of Bone and Joint Surgery, 68-A: 1041-1051.

Charnley, J. (1979). Wear of Hip Sockets. In: Low Friction Arthroplasty of the Hip (Charnley, J.). Springer-Verlag, New York, pp. 320-331.

Charnley, J. and Halley, D. K. (1975). Rate of wear in total hip replacement. Clinical Orthopaedics and Related Research, 112: 170-179.

Clarac, J. P., Pries, P., Launay, L., Martin, P., Freychet, H. and Nonet, P. (1986). Usure des cupules en polyéthylène. Etude radiologique sur 123 prosthèses totales de Charnley. Revue De Chirurgie Orthopedique Et Reparatrice De L'Appareil, 72: 97-100.

Clarke, J. C., Black, K., Rennie, C. and Amstutz, H. C. (1976). Can wear in total hip arthroplasties be assessed from radiographs? Clinical Orthopaedics and Related Research, 121: 126-142.

Collins, D. N., Chetta, S. G. and Nelson, C. L. (1982). Fracture of the acetabular cup. Journal of Bone and Joint Surgery, 64-A: 939-940.

Cupic, Z. (1979). Long term follow-up of Charnley arthroplasty of the hip. Clinical Orthopaedics and Related Research, 141: 28-43.

Johanson, N. A., Bullough, P. G., Wilson, P. D. Jr., Salvati, E. A. and Ranawat, C. S. (1987). The microscopic anatomy of the bone – cement interface in the failed total hip arthroplasties. Clinical Orthopaedics and Related Research, in press.

McCoy, T. M., Salvati, E. A., Ranawat, C. S. and Wilson, P. D. Jr. (unpublished data). A fifteen year follow-up study of one hundred Charnley low friction arthroplasties.

Moreland, J. R. and Jinnah, R. (1986). Fracture of a Charnley acetabular component from polyethylene wear. Clinical Orthopaedics and Related Research, 207: 94-96.

Muzafer, M. H. (1985). Acetabular cup fracture. <u>Orthopaedic Review,</u> 14: 546-548.


Remagen, W. and Morscher, E. (1984). Histological results with cement-free implanted hip joint sockets of polyethylene. <u>Archives of Orthopaedic and Traumatic Surgery,</u> 103: 145-151.


Rose, R. M. (1983). Materials and considerations in total hip replacement: Friction, wear and strength properties. <u>Journal of Orthopaedic Research,</u> 1: 200-201.


Rose, R. M., Nusbaum, H., Schneider, H., Ries, M., Paul, I., Crugnola, A., Simon, S. R. and Radin, E. L. (1980). On the true wear rate of ultra high molecular weight polyethylene in the total hip prosthesis. <u>Journal of Bone and Joint Surgery,</u> 62-A: 537-549.


Salvati, E. A., Wright, T. M., Burstein, A. H. and Jacobs, B. (1979). Fracture of polyethylene acetabular cups. <u>Journal of Bone and Joint Surgery,</u> 61-A: 1239-1242.


Salvati, E. A., Wilson, P. D. Jr., Jolley, M. N., Vakili, F., Aglietti, P. and Brown, G. C. (1981). A ten year follow-up of our first one hundred consecutive Charnley total hip replacements. <u>Journal of Bone and Joint Surgery,</u> 63-A: 753-767.


Stout, S. Y. and Marsh, H. O. (1981). The broken acetabular wire sign. <u>Orthopaedic Review,</u> 10: 135-137.


Willert, H. G. (1977). Reactions of the articular capsule to wear products of artificial joint prostheses. <u>Journal of Biomedical Materials Research,</u> 11: 157-164.


Wright, T. M., Burstein, A. H. and Bartel, D. L. (1985). Retrieval analysis of total joint replacement components. A six year experience. In: <u>Corrosion and Degradation of Implant Materials: Second Symposium.</u> ASTM STP 859 (Eds. Fraker, A., C. and Griffin, C. D. ), ASTM, Philadelphia, pp. 415-428.

Wroblewski, B. M. (1979).  Wear of high density polyethylene on bone and cartilage.  <u>Journal of Bone and Joint Surgery,</u> 61-B:  498-500.

Wroblewski, B. M. (1985).  Direction and rate of socket wear in Charnley low friction arthroplasty.  <u>Journal of Bone  and  Joint  Surgery,</u>  67-B: 757-761.

# 40

# ACETABULAR RECONSTRUCTION IN ARTHRITIC PATIENTS WITHOUT ACRYLIC FIXATION.

B. E. Bierbaum
S. Bogosian

## INTRODUCTION

The results from long term studies of cemented arthroplasties of the hip have shown that aseptic loosening of the acetabulum is a major problem (Charnley 1972, Salvati et al. 1981, Chandler et al. 1981, Sutherland et al. 1982). For many years, the fixation of the acetabulum with cement was considered adequate, and most concern was directed toward the femoral component (Charnley 1972, Beckenbaugh and Ilstrup 1978, Stauffer 1982, Sutherland et al. 1982). The early results of Charnley at 5 years (Charnley 1972) and 10 years (Charnley and Cupic 1973) reported revision rates of only 1·5% for the socket, whereas the 12-15 year results revealed that 25% of his acetabular sockets had either migrated (11%) or showed severe demarcation (14%).

Recent reports by Sutherland and colleagues (1982) and Stauffer (1982) both concluded that the rate of loosening of the femoral component appeared to be higher during the early follow-up period while the rate of loosening of the acetabular component appeared to be lower during the early follow-up period but increased with time. Chandler and co-authors (1981) reported on 33 hips in patients less than 30 years of age with a follow-up of 5 years. In 45% of these patients there was evidence of actual or potential loosening of the socket. The acetabular loosening occurred more than twice as frequently as femoral loosening.

The results of revision arthroplasty with bone cement are similar. Kavangh and colleagues (1985) reported on their Mayo Clinic experience of 166 hips followed both clinically and radiographically for 2 years or more. Roentgenographic analysis showed probable loosening in 20% of the acetabular components and 44% of the femoral components. The revision rate was 9%.   Pellicci and others (Pellicci et al. 1982, 1985) followed a group of 110 patients initially for between 3-8 years and then for an additional 5 years.   The initial results showed a failure rate of 14% and the later follow-up a failure rate of 29%.

Because of these reports of increasing failure rates of cemented acetabular components, we have been carrying out cementless acetabular reconstructions in both primary and revision hip replacements.   The acetabular systems used have been the Chrome-cobalt ingrowth acetabulum (Anatomic Medullary Locking), the threaded titanium ring (Mecron) and the bipolar prosthesis (Universal Hip Replacement).


## PATIENTS AND METHODS


Fifty-eight hips in 57 patients were implanted with an AML (Anatomic Medullary Locking) acetabulum with a minimum follow-up of 2 years and 6 months.   Forty-eight were implanted in "primary hips", the remaining 10 in revision cases.   The diagnoses for the primary hips were osteoarthritis in 29, inactive sepsis in 4, congenital dislocated hip in 4, slipped capital femoral epiphysis in 3, rheumatoid arthritis in 2, traumatic arthritis in 2 and haemochromatosis in 1.   The femoral prostheses utilized were the New England Baptist Stem (cementless) in 43, porous coated anatomic in 4, and New England Baptist Stem (cemented) in 1.   Acetabular grafts were carried out in 32 hips; femoral head allografts were used in 4 and autografts in 28.

The revision procedures were carried out for the following: 3 cemented loose sockets, 2 painful bipolar arthroplasties, 2 failed cementless primary arthroplasties, 1 surface replacement, 1 painful Austin-Moore prosthesis and 1 Girdlestone conversion.   At revision surgery, 2 autografts and 3 femoral head allografts were utilized, and the femoral component was revised in 9 cases.   One patient required acetabular revision due to failure of her bulk allograft.

A titanium threaded socket (Mecron) was implanted in 56 hips in 47 patients undergoing primary hip replacement and in 46 hips in 46 patients requiring revision.   The follow-up of patients undergoing a primary procedure was 9-34 months, and the underlying diagnosis was osteoarthritis in 44, rheumatoid arthritis in 5, Perthes' disease in 2, arthrodesis in 2, Marie-Strumpel disease in 1, avascular necrosis in 1 and slipped capital femoral epiphysis in 1.    During surgery, 23 acetabula required autograft.

The Mecron socket was inserted in 46 revision hips in 46 patients with a follow-up of 10–34 months.    Thirty-two revisions were performed for aseptic loosening of the acetabulum, 10 patients had had a cemented resurfacing arthroplasty, 3 had painful Austin–Moore prostheses and 1 porous coated prosthesis was converted to a threaded ring.    At surgery, 7 hips required autografts and 21 femoral head allografts.

## RESULTS

There was no evidence of lack of ingrowth or socket migration in the AML acetabula in the 48 primary procedures.    There have been 3 dislocations in 3 patients, one of whom required revision of the acetabulum to correct the instability.    The average Harris Hip Score (out of a possible 100) was 51 pre-operatively, 94 at 1 year and 96 at 2 years following surgery.

The average Harris Hip Score in the 10 revision patients was 57 pre-operatively, 82 one year post-operatively and 88 two years post-operatively.

There has been no evidence of migration or lucency of the Mecron acetabular components in the primary cases, but tangential views of the threads are difficult to obtain.    Two patients required re-operation; one socket was converted to a bipolar arthroplasty due to instability in an unco-operative octogenarian and one hip required debridement of heterotopic bone.    The Harris Hip Score averaged 57 pre-operatively and 86 post-operatively.

The following patients who had had a revisional Mecron socket required further revision operations.    A 138·6 kilogram patient had persistent pain and limp and was converted to an ingrowth socket for loosening.    Another 120·5 kilogram patient had a persistent limp following surgery.    At re-operation, his acetabulum was loose and was converted to a porous coated prosthesis.    One rheumatoid arthritic patient who had three prior total hip replacements with an incomplete acetabular ring had gross migration of the threaded socket requiring revision.    Two additional patients required re-operation to correct instability, one was revised to a bipolar arthroplasty and in the second the Mecron ring was re-aligned. The average Harris Hip Score pre-operatively was 43 and post-operatively, 80.


## DISCUSSION

In Europe, there has been more extensive experience with cementless arthroplasty and an interesting development has been the acetabular threaded device. Mittlemeier (1984a and b) reported on 432 patients implanted since 1974 with a conical screw in cup and had a 0·9% aseptic loosening rate. Gris (1984) reported on the cylindrical Lindenhof prosthesis with an average follow-up of 5 years and with an acetabular loosening rate of 8·4%. Lord's 10 year experience of 2,688 cases, in which 615 threaded ellipsoid rings were implanted, had no migrations at 5 years. Lord's current technique includes no cement with revision surgery and if the bony configuration allows a tight, contained bony socket, a threaded ring is implanted. If this cannot be achieved, a two stage procedure is planned. In the first stage, a bipolar socket is placed in the allograft; six months later, a threaded cup is implanted.

Our results with the threaded cup in primary and revision hip surgery are similar to those reported in the literature. Our primary hip procedures show no evidence of migration or of loose fixation. However, in two groups of patients undergoing revisional surgery the prosthesis has failed; 2 overweight patients and one patient with rheumatoid arthritis and an incomplete bony acetabulum had unsuccessful revisonal surgery with the threaded ring.

The bipolar cup has been used for primary as well as revisional surgery. Much of the clinical experience has come from its use following displaced femoral neck fractures. The acetabular deterioration encountered with the Austin-Moore and Thompson prostheses eventually led to its design. The results of the bipolar prosthesis for osteoarthritis or rheumatoid arthritis are described elsewhere in this Festschrift (p. 256). However, it still remains to be proven whether the bipolar socket is an alternative when intact articular cartilage is present.

Satisfactory results have been achieved in revisional surgery with a bipolar prosthesis supplemented with allograft. Five mm. in diameter pieces of bone are obtained from the allograft femoral head and packed into the deficient acetabulum. The packing is facilitated by using conventional socket reamers in reverse rotation. This process is repeated until the acetabulum is at the anatomic location. Following allograft preparation, the bipolar head prosthesis is implanted. Rim contact between the bipolar and host acetabula is essential to prevent migration. Bulk graft may be utilized in certain cases of rim deficiency, and with it a bipolar prosthesis or a porous coated prosthesis has yielded successful early results. We are impressed with the apparent incorporation of the allograft to host bone as demonstrated on conventional x-rays.

We use the bipolar prosthesis when there is intact articular cartilage, and combined with massive allografting in the deficient acetabulum requiring bone replacement. The threaded ring has been ideal for protrusio and patients with intact acetabular bone stock. We caution its use in revision surgery if the bone stock is inadequate or if the patient is of excessive weight. The combination of threaded socket and porous ingrowth socket deserves evaluation for revision surgery. Theoretically, the hemispherical porous coated socket may be the most durable acetabulum, but long term studies of at least 10 year follow-up are required to evaluate the cementless acetabulum.

## REFERENCES

Beckenbaugh, R. D. and Ilstrup, D. M. (1978). Total hip arthroplasty. A review of three hundred and thirty-three cases with long-term follow-up. Journal of Bone and Joint Surgery, 60-A: 306-313.

Chandler, H. P., Reineck, F. T., Wilson, R. L. and McCarthy, J. C. (1982). Total hip replacement in patients younger than thirty years old. A five year follow-up study. Journal of Bone and Joint Surgery, 63-A: 1426-1434.

Charnley, J. (1972). The long-term results of low friction arthroplasty of the hip performed as a primary intervention. Journal of Bone and Joint Surgery, 54-B: 61-76.

Charnley, J. and Cupic, Z. (1973). The nine and ten year results of the low-friction arthroplasty of the hip. Clinical Orthopaedics and Related Research, 95: 9-25.

Charnley, J. (1979). Low Friction Arthroplasty of the Hip. Springer-Verlag, Berlin.

Gris (1984). Four to eight year post-operative results of partially uncemented Lidenholf-type ceramic hip endoprosthesis. In: The Cementless Fixation of Hip Endoprosthesis. Springer-Verlag, pp. 220-224.

Kavangh, B., Ilstrup, D. M. and Fitzgerald, R. H. (1985). Revision total hip arthroplasty. Journal of Bone and Joint Surgery, 67-A: 517-526.

Mittlemeier, H. (1984a). Eight years of experience with self-locking ceramic hip prosthesis "Autophor". Journal of Bone and Joint Surgery, 66-B: 300.

Mittlemeier, H. (1984b). Total hip replacement with the Autophor cement-free ceramic prosthesis. In: The Cementless Fixation of Hip Endoprosthesis. Springer-Verlag, pp. 225-241.

Pellicci, P., Wilson, P. D., Sledge, C. B., Salvati, E. A., Ranawat, C. S. and Poss, R. (1982). Revision total hip arthroplasty. Clinical Orthopaedics and Related Research, 170: 34-41.

Pellicci, P., Wilson, P. D., Sledge, C. B., Salvati, E. A., Ranawat, C. S., Poss, R. and Callaghan, J. J. (1985). Long term results of revision total hip replacement. Journal of Bone and Joint Surgery, 67-A: 513-516.

Salvati, E. A., Wilson, P. D., Jolley, M. N. Vakali, F., Aghetti, P. and Brown G. C. (1981). A ten year follow-up study of our first one hundred consecutive Charnley total hip replacements. Journal of Bone and Joint Surgery, 63-A: 753-767.

Stauffer, R. N. (1982). Ten year follow-up study of total hip replacement: with particular reference to roentgenographic loosening of the components. Journal of Bone and Joint Surgery, 64-A: 983-990.

Sutherland, C. J., Wilde, A. H., Borden, L. S. and Marks, K. E. (1982). A ten year follow-up of one hundred consecutive Muller curved-stem total hip replacement arthroplasties. Journal of Bone and Joint Surgery, 64-A: 970-982.

41.

# APPLICATION OF A MULTIPLE BEARING IMPLANT IN HIP JOINT RECONSTRUCTION – A 10-YEAR ANALYSIS OF 1007 CASES, INCLUDING THE USE OF AUTOGENOUS CEMENT.

J. E. Bateman

A bipolar type of implant has been used over a 10 year period in 1007 instances for hip reconstruction (Figures 1 and 2). The multiple bearing concept was introduced in 1973 and used initially for fractures in the elderly, aseptic necrosis, non-union, and some osteo-arthritic patients (Bateman 1977). It subsequently has been used in a much greater range of problems (Lestrange 1979, West and Mann 1979, Long and Knight 1980, Schildhaus 1980, VanDemark et al. 1980), including revision of hemi- and total arthroplasties. The hemi-arthroplasties were revised

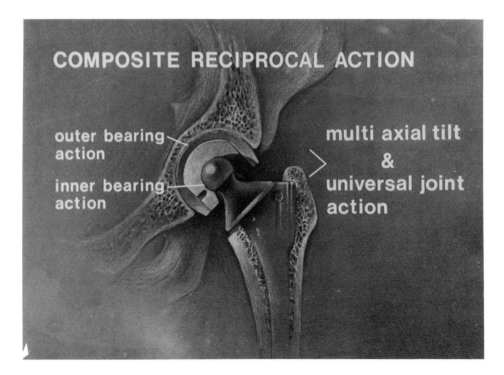

FIG. 1.    Diagrammatic representation of the multiple bearing action.

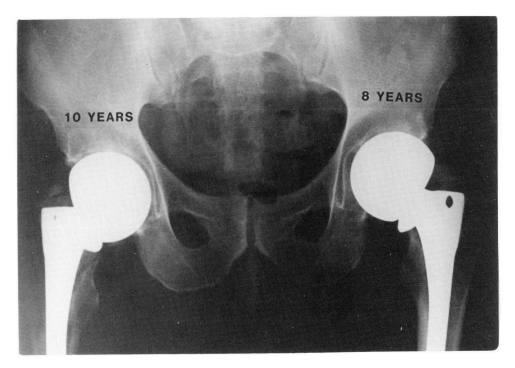

FIG. 2.    Bilateral bipolar arthroplasties carried out 10 years  (right) and 8 years (left) previously for bilateral osteo-arthritis.

for  pelvic  floor  protrusion  or  ectopic  bone  formation.   Where the acetabular component of a total hip arthroplasty was firmly  fixed  only the femoral component was revised.   If a 22 mm. cup had previously been inserted the polyethylene was reamed with a high speed  burr  to  accept the  smallest  diameter head.    This paper describes the results in these patients.

The Harris method of scoring has been used routinely.   The follow-up assessment  was carried out by physiotherapists (Mode and Thornton 1978) with clinicians  checking the patients and records.   The patients  were assessed  at  discharge  from hospital and at 6 months.   The first  453 patients  were  assessed  at  yearly  intervals  for  5  years  and  the survivors were again assessed at 10 years.

RESULTS

The  results  obtained  in  all  the  patients  are  shown  in  Table I.

| | PRE-OPERATIVE | |
| --- | --- | --- |
| | RANGE | AVERAGE |
| Unilateral osteo-arthritis (441 hips)<br>Age Range 31–86<br>Average 62·77 | 15–70 | 50·7 |
| Bilateral osteo-arthritis (164 hips)<br>Age Range 51–78<br>Average 64·47 | 23–85 | 45·6 |
| Rheumatoid Arthritis (82 hips)<br>Age Range 34–74<br>Average 54·42 | 30–71 | 43 |
| Arthrodesis and Ankylosis (70 hips)<br>Age Range 33–82<br>Average 60·28 | 19–78 | 45 |
| Failed Cup Arthroplasty (66 hips)<br>Age Range 43–74<br>Average 59·7 | 15–76 | 49·8 |
| Failed Hemi-arthroplasty (49 hips)<br>Age Range 32–84<br>Average 67·4 | 43–69 | 51·5 |
| Fractures (34 hips)<br>Age Range 78–94<br>Average 85 | – | – |
| Congenital Dislocation of the Hip (44 hips)<br>Age Range 38–54<br>Average 46·5 | 22–53 | 42·2 |
| Aseptic Necrosis (12 hips)<br>Age Range 27–59<br>Average 54 | 40–70 | 51 |
| Failed Total Arthroplasty (45 hips)<br>Age Range 44–78<br>Average 66 | 26–45 | 33·3 |
| Protrusio Acetabuli (10 hips)<br>Age Range 28–72<br>Average 54·3 | 29–72 | 53·6 |

I
SURGICAL INDICATION
HIPS

| | 6 MONTHS POST-OPERATIVE | AVERAGE INCREMENT AT 6 MONTHS |
| RANGE | AVERAGE | |
| --- | --- | --- |
| 85–100 | 87 | 30·7 |
| 65–100 | 82·4 | 36·8 |
| 78–100 | 82 | 39 |
| 78–100 | 82 | 37 |
| 60–97 | 82·3 | 32·5 |
| 55–99 | 84·9 | 33·4 |
| 60–84 | 72 | – |
| 62–96 | 74·6 | 32·4 |
| 78–84 | 82 | 31 |
| 58–93 | 79·4 | 46·1 |
| 55–95 | 81·1 | 26.8 |

Irrespective of the indication for surgery there was an improvement in all the patients. The greatest change occurred in those patients who had a failed total hip arthroplasty.

The results of the 5 annual assessments in the first 453 patients are shown in Table II. In general terms their improvement was maintained during this period.

The overall complication rates in all patients are shown in Table III.

A group of 130 successive patients who were operated upon in 1973, 1974 and 1975, and in whom 149 hips had been operated upon were studied at the end of 5 and 10 years. One hundred and six patients were available for review at 5 years, 89 of whom had retained a score of 80 to 100. Fifty patients were available for assessment at the end of 10 years. Forty-five claimed 100% relief of pain and could walk further than at the time of surgery. Forty-four were classified as good to excellent. Revisions had been required in 3. Three patients complained of shortening and 5 had developed joint disease affecting their contralateral hip.

The one specific complication related to this implant was disassembly (Anderson and Milgram 1978, Barmada and Siegel 1979). In two instances the inner bearing fractured through one of the leaves allowing the femoral component to dislocate. This complication occurred 4 and 5 years respectively after surgery in heavily built patients, following strenuous lower limb activity. Replacement with a bipolar implant has been followed by an uncomplicated course in both instances.

Slight sinking of the femoral head into the acetabulum was common in osteoporotic rheumatoid patients receiving steroids and in two instances revision using a larger head was required at 5 years with satisfactory stability being obtained.

Five of the 10 patients who had surgery for protrusio acetabuli developed thickening of their acetabular floor.


## DISCUSSION

The results of this study confirm that a single assembly type of total implant can be used in a wide variety of arthropathies of the hip joint

TABLE II

LONG TERM RESULTS (HARRIS SCORE)

MONTHS POST-OPERATIVE

| INDICATION | PRE-OP | DISCHARGE | 6 | 12 | 24 | 36 | 48 | 60 |
|---|---|---|---|---|---|---|---|---|
| Unilateral osteo-arthritis | 59 | 81 | 100 | 100 | 100 | 100 | 95 | 100 |
| Bilateral osteo-arthritis – Right | 54 | 70 | 86 | 95 | 99 | 98 | 100 | 98 |
| – Left | 56 | 74 | 98 | 98 | 98 | 95 | 100 | 97 |
| Rheumatoid arthritis | 65 | 83 | 91 | 91 | 91 | 91 | 91 | 91 |
| Arthrodesis and ankylosis | 32 | 77 | 98 | 100 | 99 | 100 | 99 | 99 |
| Failed cup arthroplasty | 46 | 62 | 67 | 84 | 92 | 92 | 93 | 95 |
| Failed hemi-arthroplasty | 50 | 56 | 79 | 83 | 93 | 99 | 99 | 99 |
| Fractures | – | 85 | 90 | 96 | 96 | 100 | 97 | 97 |
| Congenital dislocation of the hip | 48 | 70 | 78 | 90 | 92 | 90 | 90 | 90 |
| Aseptic necrosis | 47 | 70 | 92 | 95 | 100 | 100 | 100 | 100 |
| Failed total arthroplasty | 44 | 66 | 78 | 80 | 85 | 92 | 85 | 85 |
| Protrusio acetabuli | 59 | 75 | 83 | 95 | 96 | 96 | 96 | 96 |

with preservation of the acetabulum. The clinical improvement observed at six months has been retained over a 10 year span in a uniform fashion. The implant can be inserted with relatively little technical difficulty in most hip deformities. It also can be used without methyl methacrylate. The last 400 implants, of whom 225 were in patients aged 55 or younger, were inserted without methyl methacrylate and in the most recent 270 instances a cancellous "mash" was packed into the femoral canal in place of the methyl methacrylate. The femoral head was curretted with a high speed burr and autogenous plasma added to the mixture (Rhinelander et al. 1979). The plasma was prepared as a cancellous adhesive by cold centrifuging 50 cc. of the patient's blood beforehand. The plasma was mixed with the cancellous grafts, and coagulation was obtained by adding topical thrombin to produce a

TABLE III

| COMPLICATION | NUMBER | | PER CENT |
|---|---|---|---|
| Infection | | | |
| Wound seepage with positive culture | 20 | ) | |
| | | ) | 2·7% |
| Persistent wound infection* | 7 | ) | |
| Phlebitis | 3 | | 0.29% |
| Pulmonary embolism | 2 | | 0·19% |
| Dislocation | | | |
| Early: 0-21 days | 3 | | 0·3% |
| Late:  0-84 months | 3 | | 0.3% |
| Disassembly | 2 | | 0·2% |

* 5 had previous osteomyelitis

jelly-like mass.    The  shaft was tightly packed so that when the stem was inserted it literally had to be hammered  into  place  providing  an extremely  strong  method of fixation.    In 42 patients scintigraphy was used to evaluate  the  osteogenic  potential  of  the  cancellous  mash. There  was evidence of vascularisation starting at 7 days and continuing for 11 weeks.

In some instances such as in protrusio acetabuli the configuration of the  acetabular  floor  has improved following insertion of the implant. The implant is not presented as a panacea for all  types  of  hip  joint abnormality  but  the experience obtained to date indicates that it is a useful  addition  to  the  procedures  available  for  hip  joint reconstruction.

REFERENCES

Anderson,    R.   and  Milgram,   W.   (1978).    Dislocation  and  component separation of the Bateman hip endoprosthesis.  Journal of  the  American Medical Association, 240:  2079-2080.

Barmada,   R. and Siegel, I. M. (1979).   Post-operative separation of the femoral  and  acetabular  components  of  a  single  assembly  total  hip (Bateman)  replacement:   Report  of 2 cases.   Journal of Bone and Joint

Surgery, 61-A:   777-778.


Bateman, E. (1977). Experiences with a multiple-bearing implant in reconstruction for hip deformities. Orthopaedic Transactions, 1:   242.


Lestrange, N. R. (1979). The Bateman UPF prosthesis:   A 48 month experience. Orthopaedics, 2:   182-186.


Long, J. W. and Knight, W. H. (1980). Bateman UPF prosthesis in fractures of the femoral neck. Clinical Orthopaedics and Related Research, 152:   198-201.


Mode, M. and Thornton, S. (1978). Rehabilitation and the hip following single assembly total hip replacement. Physiotherapy Canada, 30:  291-294.


Rhinelander, F. W., Nelson, C. L., Stewart, R. D. and Stewart, C. L. (1979). Experimental reaming of the proximal femur and acrylic cement implantation:   Vascular and histological effects. In: Proceedings of the 7th Open Scientific Meeting of the Hip Society, p. 127.


Schildhaus, S. E. (1980). The Bateman universal proximal femoral assembly:   Experience with 80 cases. Orthopaedics, 3:   974-980.


VanDemark, R. E. Jr., Cabanela, M. E. and Henderson, E. D. (1980). The Bateman endoprosthesis:   104 arthroplasties. Orthopaedic Transactions, 4:   356.


West, W. F. and Mann, R. A. (1979). Evaluation of the Bateman self-articulating femoral prosthesis. Orthopaedic Transactions, 3:   17.

# 42

# THE USE OF STANDARDIZED RADIOGRAPHS TO IDENTIFY THE DEFORMITIES ASSOCIATED WITH OSTEOARTHRITIS

T. D. V. Cooke
D. Siu
B. Fisher

## INTRODUCTION

The association between abnormalities of joint surfaces and osteoarthritis is well defined. Thus, at the hip, the dysplastic configuration of the joint carries a well defined incidence of superolateral osteoarthritis (Lloyd-Roberts 1955, Hely et al. 1984). Likewise, at the knee, Blount's disease leads to a significant incidence of medial compartment osteoarthritis in adult life. Nonetheless, a wide variety of varus or valgus knees do not develop osteoarthritis. Whilst the correlation between osteoarthritis and excessive mechanical stress is very well defined (Radin 1976), it is not absolute. Other factors, including a systemic disposition for polyarthritis (Kellgren et al. 1963), inflammatory or immune changes (Cooke 1986), and crystal deposition disease (Dieppe et al. 1978) may all act as risk or accelerating factors. It. has been suggested that most cases of osteoarthritis represent the interaction of at least two or more such factors (Cooke 1985).

The observation of progressive medial compartment osteoarthritis in patients with an inward sloping joint in the coronal plane (excessive distal femoral valgus and tibia vara) was first reported in 1985 (Cooke and Pichora 1985). These knee dysplasias had a medialized load bearing axis and marked lateral tibial subluxation. The incidence of this problem was unknown. The aim of this study was to define the incidence of dysplastic knees in a random consecutive population of patients with arthritis of the knee referred to our orthopaedic clinics.

## MATERIALS, METHODS AND PATIENTS

The data were derived from analysis of radiographs of 220 consecutive patients to three orthopaedic surgeons at Kingston General Hospital from 1981 to 1985 (Table 1).    All patients had a standardized radiographic assessment of both knees.    In 18% of patients, knee surgery (osteotomy or a replacement) was carried out.    These patients were entered into a prospective study for future data analysis.

### TABLE 1.

Demographic data of the osteoarthritic patients.

| Sex | Number of patients | Age Range (Mean) | Incidence of Bilaterality Number of Patients | % of Knees |
|---|---|---|---|---|
| Male | 82 | 41–83 (64) | 23 | 21 |
| Female | 138 | 29–88 (68) | 35 | 32 |

Standing, antero-posterior and lateral orthogonal radiographs were taken to assess knee alignment (Wevers et al. 1982).    In essence, the patient stood in a frame on a rotating platform with the ankles set against markers on the platform.    The hips and knees were aligned and tibial rotation assessed by the position of the second toe on radians marked on the rotating platform.    Antero-posterior radiographs were taken of both knees and hips using cassettes held in the frame behind the patient.    The patient was rotated precisely 90° to left or right respectively without any change in knee position, and a lateral orthogonal view of each knee obtained.

Landmarks of the femur, proximal tibia and hip were identified on each film, and these, plus the radiographic markers, were digitized using a digitizing tablet (Science Accessories Corporation).    The recorded data was stored in a personal computer (Zenith Data Systems Corporation) and were displayed as a series of numeric values for dimensional and angular data of each knee with a diagrammatic outline of the hip, knee, and ankle alignment (stick diagram – Figure 1).    This technique has a laboratory precision of better than 1 mm. and 1° (Wevers et al. 1982), but standard errors of the mean up to 2 mm. in geometric assessment and 2° in alignment have been observed in the clinic.

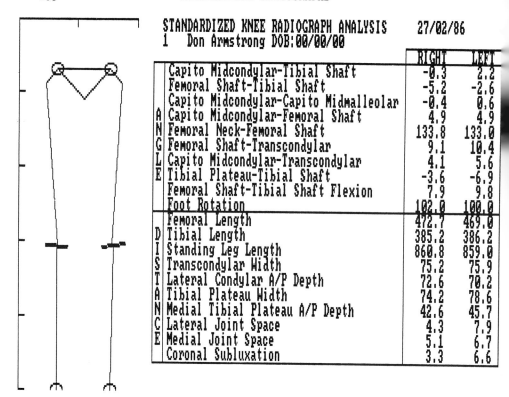

FIG. 1.   Sample  of  a  computerized  output  of  angular  and  linear
dimensional parameters with a diagrammatic outline  (stick  diagram)  of
the lower limbs.

The  angular  orientation of bony parts of the knee to each other varied
in different clinical groups.    Therefore,  a  standardized  nomenclature
was  developed (Figures 1 and 2).    The capito midcondylar-transcondylar
angle represented the relationship of the tangents of the knee articular
surface to the hip (Figure 2a) and the femoral shaft-transcondylar angle
represented its relationship to the femoral shaft (Figure 2b).

     The data was analysed with software programme known as SYSTAT.


## RESULTS


The overall pattern in  osteoarthritis  showed  deviation  of  the  load
bearing  angle (LBA) medially in two thirds (varus knees), and laterally
in one third (valgus knees).    Twenty one per cent  were  within  2°  of
neutral alignment (no significant deformity).

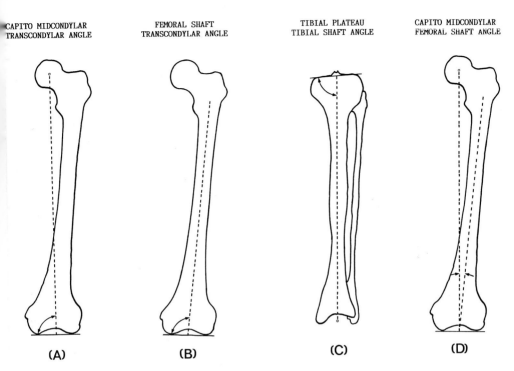

| CAPITO MIDCONDYLAR TRANSCONDYLAR ANGLE | FEMORAL SHAFT TRANSCONDYLAR ANGLE | TIBIAL PLATEAU TIBIAL SHAFT ANGLE | CAPITO MIDCONDYLAR FEMORAL SHAFT ANGLE |
|---|---|---|---|
| (A) | (B) | (C) | (D) |

FIG. 2. Details of the angular orientation made by the tangents of the knee articular surfaces to the hip, femoral shaft and ankle.

Figure 3 is a representation of all the knees. Males are shown as single solid squares and females as open squares. On the vertical axis, are plotted the variation in varus (–) or valgus (+) of the tibial surface from the right angle to the ankle (the zero axis). On the horizontal axis, the variation of the transcondylar tangent beyond the right angle to the hip has been plotted (– varus, + valgus). The zero intercepts represent a limb in which the tibial margins are at a right angle to the ankle with the femoral surfaces at a right angle to the hip.

Femoral alignment

There was a preponderance of knees with tibia vara and a valgus capito midcondylar-transcondylar angle (a valgus orientation of the distal femur to the hip). A valgus femoral orientation to the hip was present in 85% with the maximal deviation being +14°. The incidence of dysplastic femora (a capito midcondylar-transcondylar valgus more than 3°) was surprisingly high – it was seen in 45% of all patients. The excessive valgus femur (dysplastic) was associated with tibia vara in

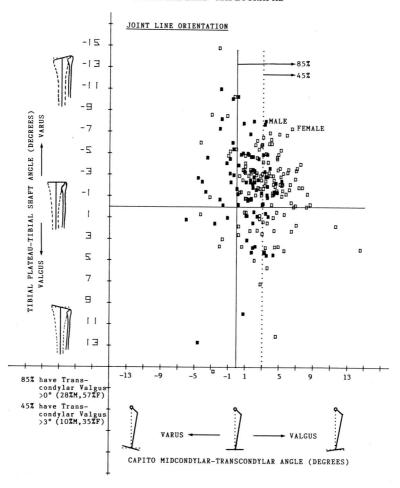

FIG. 3.    Graphic  representation  of osteoarthritic knees:  a plot of
tibial        plateau–tibial        shaft        angle        versus        capito
midcondylar–transcondylar angle.   Varus (– ve) and valgus (+ ve).

34%.


Tibial alignment

The  tibial geometry revealed a range of deformity from 15° varus to 13°
valgus.    The  mean  was  2°  varus,  correlating  with  the  overall
medialization  of  knee  alignment  in the majority.    However, when the
neutral tibia was associated with excessive valgus of the femur  to  the
femoral  head,  an  overall  valgus  deformity  was  produced.    These 47
patients exemplify the "valgus form" of knee  dysplasia.    In  22,  the
lateral  compartment, rather than medial compartment, showed predominant
arthritis.

Relationship between differences in joint space (medial-lateral compartment) to load bearing axis

There was a broad correlation between relatively greater medial or lateral joint space loss and varus or valgus knee alignment respectively. However, an unexpected incidence of mismatched data was found. Thus, lateral joint space loss occurred in varus knees and vice versa. In the 7 varus mismatched knees, a femoral dysplasia of more than 3° was found in 6. Likewise, in the 47 valgus knees with medial joint space loss, the incidence of excessive valgus of the femur (dysplastic) to the hip was found in 45 cases.

Relationship between capito midcondylar-transcondylar valgus and femoral shaft transcondylar valgus (Figure 2d).

In 92% of knees, the angular orientation of the femoral bearing surface to the hip varied in a direct and proportional relationship to the shaft. In this arthritic population, the capito midcondylar-transcondylar valgus mean was 2·5°. These data imply that the angular orientation between the shaft, the mechanical axis and the femoral head varied little. This was indeed the case; a narrow angle of between 4° and 7° was found with a mean of 5·6°.


DISCUSSION


One purpose of this study was to evaluate the incidence of dysplastic knees in osteoarthritis. The findings revealed an unexpectedly high incidence of dysplasia which, in retrospect, clearly related to the radiographic capability to detect this condition. Without a way to define and measure the femoral condylar tangent orientation to the hip joint, the excessively valgus dysplastic femur is easily missed. The generally accepted range of angular orientation of the distal femur to the hip varied between 5° and 10° (Hood and Insall 1984). Our results showed that 45% of these knees were in excess of this figure with a valgus orientation of >3° to hip. We found no evidence for a relationship between distal femoral orientation and the hip, but there was an extremely high correlation to the valgus orientation to the shaft. This means that in the general population, the variation of shaft to knee to hip alignment is small. In this osteoarthritic population a range of 4° to 7°, with a mean of 5·6°, was found.

In our clinical assessment of dysplastic osteoarthritic knees, we initially screened patients with a distal femoral valgus of greater than 10°, but the results of this study suggest that any angular orientation over 7° may be considered abnormal. The varus dysplastic knee, with a capito midcondylar-transcondylar valgus of more than 3°, was found in 45% of patients. The medialized load bearing axis producing the varus knee, was produced by a combination of tibia vara and medial joint space collapse. Among the valgus osteoarthritic knees, the dysplastic femur was implicated in 63%. Here, the neutral tibial orientation allowed for an overall lateralization of the load bearing axis. In the majority of these patients, lateral joint compartment osteoarthritis predominated over medial.

The implications of the dysplastic knee are not dealt with in detail in this study, but our analysis in specific cases suggested that these deformed knees carry a high risk of lateral tibial and patella subluxation and rapidly progressive arthritis (Cooke and Pichora – in preparation). Our analysis further suggested that the dysplastic angular aberration of distal femoral and proximal tibial surfaces was often in more than one plane. In the varus dysplastic knee, the rotational aberrations tended to vary in opposite directions for the distal femur and proximal tibia respectively. Thus, the distal femur tended to twist inwards about its long axis and outwards in the coronal plane, whereas there was an outward twist of the upper tibia about its long axis and a varus alignment to the ankle. The net result was an inward sloping joint line with proximal distal axial rotations in opposite plane.

These data have important implications for surgery. Knees suitable for osteotomy, with mainly single joint compartment changes, must be carefully assessed for the extent of femoral dysplasia. In the varus knee, with a femoral condylar tangent within a few degrees of the right angle to the hip an upper tibial osteotomy is highly logical. However, in the varus dysplastic knee, the medial compartment osteoarthritis of the varus knee is inadequately treated by upper tibial osteotomy alone. We use a varus distal femoral osteotomy to correct the excessive femoral valgus and then a valgus upper tibial osteotomy to bring the load bearing axis lateral to the knee. Our aim is to bring the inwards slanting knee joint closer to the horizontal. Osteotomy for lateral compartment osteoarthritis in the valgus dysplastic knee requires a varus femoral osteotomy alone since the tibia is usually in neutral (Coventry 1973, Shoji and Insall 1973).

In total knee arthroplasty, placement of the components must **not** be referenced to the excessively valgus and inwardly rotated medial condyles. We use the transverse axis of the epicondyles to define neutral rotation of the femur and reference femoral component placement to this. Lack of recognition of the dysplastic configuration, in the varus or valgus knee, easily leads to malplaced components (usually in excess valgus and internal rotation) with a continuing tendency for lateral tibial subluxation and lateral patella dislocation. Obliquity may be a cause of tibial subluxation in the varus knee and we agree with others that the components should be placed at a right angle to the load bearing axis in total knee replacement (Hood and Install 1984, Clayton et al. 1986).

Many questions remain unanswered by this study. The relevance of discrepancies in data between medial joint space loss and valgus knee alignment, and vice versa, as well as characterization of rotary abnormalities of the femur and tibia respectively, await further study.

The results of this study indicate that a standardized method for assessing the knee in stance is of great value, both to allow accurate identification of the dysplastic configuration and to analyse the variations in geometry of the femur and tibia. The data suggests that malformations of the knee may be a risk factor in the development of osteoarthritis, and that the dysplastic excessively valgus distal femur is commonly implicated.

## ACKNOWLEDGEMENTS

The authors wish to acknowledge the support and help of other members of the CMG, the Radiology staff at Kingston General Hospital, especially Mrs. Linda McKinven, and the diligent typing skills of Lee Watkins.

Technical References

GrafPen GP-6-30 ZD Digitizer

Science Accessories Corporation,

970, King's Highway West,

Southport, Connecticut 06490, UNITED STATES OF AMERICA.

Zenith ZW-158-42
Zenith Data Systems Corporation,
Saint Joseph, Michigan 49085, UNITED STATES OF AMERICA.

Systat The System for Statistics
Systat Incorporated,
603, Main Street,
Evanston, Illinois 60202, UNITED STATES OF AMERICA.

## REFERENCES

Clayton, M., Thompson, T. R. and Mack, R. P. (1986). Correction of alignment deformities during total knee arthroplasties: Staged soft-tissue releases. Clinical Orthopaedics and Related Research, 202: 117-124.

Cooke, T. D. V. (1985). Pathogenetic mechanisms in polyarticular osteoarthritis. Clinics in Rheumatic Diseases, 11: 203-238.

Cooke, T. D. V. (1986). Immune pathology in polyarticular osteoarthritis. Clinical Orthopaedics and Related Research, 213: 41-49.

Cooke, T. D. V. and Pichora, D. (1985). Knee dysplasia: An unusual but important problem associated with progressive arthritis. Journal of Bone and Joint Surgery, 67-B: 332.

Cooke, T. D. V. and Pichora, D. (in preparation). Abnormalities of articular surface alignment and their relationship to arthritis of the knee joint. I. The varus forms of knee dysplasia.

Coventry, M. B. (1973). Osteotomy about the knee for degenerative and rheumatoid arthritis. Indications of operative technique and results. Journal of Bone and Joint Surgery, 55-A: 23-48.

Dieppe, P. A., Doyle, D. V., Huskisson, E. C., Willoughby, D. A. and Crocker, P. R. (1978). Mixed crystal deposition disease and osteoarthritis. British Medical Journal, 1: 150.

Hely, D. P., Salvati, E. A. and Pellicci, P. M. (1984). The Hip. In: Adult Orthopaedics. (Eds. Cruess, R. L. and Rennie, W. R. J.), Churchill Livingstone, New York, Volume 2, pp. 1209-1274.

Hood, R. W. and Insall, J. N. (1984). The Knee. In: Adult Orthopaedics. (Eds. Cruess, R. L. and Rennie, W. R. J.), Churchill Livingstone, New York, Volume 2, pp. 1275-1406.

Kellgren, J. H., Lawrence, J. S. and Bier, F. (1963). Genetic factors in generalized osteoarthritis. Annals of the Rheumatic Diseases, 22: 237-255.

Lloyd-Roberts, G. C. (1955). Osteoarthritis: A study of the clinical pathology. Journal of Bone and Joint Surgery, 37-B: 8-47.

Radin, E. L. (1976). Mechanical aspects of osteoarthritis. Bulletin of the Rheumatic Diseases, 26: 862-865.

Shoji, H. and Insall, J. (1973). High tibial osteotomy for osteoarthritis of the knee with valgus deformity. Journal of Bone and Joint Surgery, 55-A: 963-973.

Wevers, H. W., Siu, D. W. and Cooke, T. D. V. (1982). A quantitative method of assessing malalignment of joint space loss of the human knee. Journal of Biomedical Engineering, 4: 319-324.

# 43

# THE TOTAL CONDYLAR KNEE REPLACEMENT – A ROBUST AND RELIABLE PROSTHESIS

J. Noble
J. P. Hodgkinson
K. J. Drabu
H. Potts

## INTRODUCTION

Attempts to match the normal anatomy of the joint with conservation of bone, correction of soft tissue imbalance, and patellar resurfacing has resulted in the development of the semi-constrained yet unlinked prostheses such as the total condylar knee prosthesis (Insall et al. 1979). Previous designs such as the semi-constrained or linked prosthesis had been associated with a high incidence of loosening.

Previously reported results of the total condylar knee replacement showed that excellent pain relief was achieved in 95% of knees with a 2 year follow-up (Scott and Volatile 1986) and 87·5% of knees remained satisfactory after 10 years (Insall et al. 1986). There has been no similar study from the United Kingdom. The impression received from a number of centres is that the results of knee replacement may be as favourable as those of hip replacement surgery, and this study was carried out to determine our results.

## PATIENTS AND METHODS

Between January 1980 and September 1986, 177 total condylar knee prostheses have been implanted in 153 patients. The procedures were performed mainly by the senior author (J.N.) although a small number were carried out by members of the junior staff under his supervision. A total of 166 knees (Group A) in 143 patients have been reviewed by an independent observer (J.P.H.). Five of the other 10 patients (with 11 knee arthroplasties) had died of unrelated causes and 5 could not be traced as their hospital records were missing.

One hundred and twenty-six arthroplasties (Group B) in 108 patients with a minimum follow-up of 2 years (average 3·5 years) have been reassessed in terms of pain, function, range of movement and radiographic alignment.

Many of the operations had been carried out in operating theatres shared with general surgeons, and without laminar airflow facilities. The procedure was performed under tourniquet through a mid-line anterior incision, although occasionally a previous scar had to be used. Appropriate ligament and soft tissue releases were made before any bone cuts were performed. The bone cuts were made using the original 3 Insall instruments and checked with the alignment rods. An appropriately sized prosthesis was selected and in all cases the patella was resurfaced. Antibiotic-loaded acrylic cement was used and the wound was closed, after lateral release of the patella where indicated.

Post-operatively, the patients were nursed in a wool and crepe bandage and removable splint. The drains were removed at 48 hours and the patient allowed to mobilize weight-bearing in the splint. Quadriceps exercises were commenced from day 1, and on day 5, if the wound was satisfactory, gentle knee flexion exercises were commenced. Attempts to improve knee flexion by manipulation under anaesthesia were largely abandoned after the first year, as this had been shown not to improve long term results (Fox and Poss 1981).

## RESULTS

The average age of the 143 patients was 65·3 years (range 32 to 82 years) and there were 36 males and 107 females. The pre-operative diagnosis was rheumatoid arthritis in 112 knees (67·5%) and osteoarthritis in 54 (32·5%). In all patients the main indication for surgery was severe pre-operative pain, which included rest and night pain.

Pre-operative radiographic assessment revealed a valgus deformity in 64 knees (range 3 – 40°, average 17°) and a varus deformity in 56 knees (range 3 – 35°, average 14°); 6 knees were in neutral. Thirty knees (17%) had undergone previous surgery (Table 1), the commonest operation being upper tibial osteotomy (9 knees) and previous arthroplasty (7 knees).

Table 1

The number and type of operations performed prior to total condylar replacement (Group A).

| PREVIOUS SURGERY | NUMBER OF PATIENTS |
|---|---|
| Medial meniscectomy | 5 |
| Lateral meniscectomy | 1 |
| Tibial osteotomy | 9 |
| Synovectomy | 3 |
| Patellectomy | 1 |
| Arthroplasty | 7 |
| Arthrotomy and debridement | 4 |
| Arthroscopy | 3 |
| TOTAL | 33 |

Complications

The overall complication rate following 166 knee arthroplasties (Group A) was 26·5%. This included 10 patients (6%) who suffered systemic complications (Table 2). There were no immediate (within 3 months) post-operative deaths.

Table 2

The systemic post-operative complications.

| COMPLICATIONS | NUMBER |
|---|---|
| Deep vein thrombosis | 4 |
| Pulmonary embolism | 2 |
| Myocardial infarction | 2 |
| Renal failure | 1 |
| Acute urinary retention | 1 |
| TOTAL | 10 |

The other post-operative complications are shown in Table 3.

## Table 3

The local post-operative complications.

| COMPLICATIONS | NUMBER |
|---|---|
| Superficial infection | 6 |
| Deep infection (early) | 0 |
| Deep infection (late) | 2 |
| Delayed wound healing (> 3 weeks) | 23 |
| Fractured patella | 1 |
| Patella ligament rupture | 1 |
| Common peroneal nerve palsy | 3 |
| Revision required | 3 |
| TOTAL | 39 |

### Superficial infections

Six patients developed minor, superficial wound infections from which staphylococcus epidermidis or "scanty skin flora" were isolated. All were treated by immobilization and daily dressings, and 4 patients were also given an appropriate antibiotic. All healed fully and none have developed any further signs of infection.

### Deep infections

There were no early deep infections but 2 patients developed a late infection, more than 18 months after surgery. Both patients were male, osteoarthritic and gave a history of a fall down stairs injuring their knee arthroplasty, whilst they had an upper respiratory tract infection. In both patients the organism was staphylococcus aureus, and both required arthrodesis.

### Delayed wound healing

Twenty-three wounds took longer than 3 weeks to heal and of these, 5 required some plastic surgical procedure to achieve successful skin cover. Three of these patients had rheumatoid arthritis and were taking steroids and/or penicillamine. The other 2 patients had osteoarthritis; 2 had had previous surgery and one was diabetic. All 5 patients subsequently did well and regained at least 90° of flexion.

Prosthetic loosening

One knee was successfully revised for aseptic loosening of the tibial component.

Peroneal nerve palsy

Peroneal nerve palsy occurred in 3 patients associated with correction of fixed valgus deformities. All 3 recovered spontaneously and totally; the first within an hour, the second in 6 weeks and the third within 3 months.

Patellar problems

One patient, who suffered a fractured patella in a fall, was treated by open reduction and internal fixation and recovered satisfactorily. One dysvascular patient who had undergone several previous operations to the knee suffered a gradual rupture of the patellar ligament, but she was painfree and able to mobilize in a knee brace, having refused the option of repair.

Pain relief, and functional results

In the 126 knees (Group B) with a minimum 2 year follow-up, complete pain relief was achieved in 103 (81·7%) and a further 19 (15·1%) had only occasional, mild pain on walking (Table 4). Only 4 patients (3·2%) had unsatisfactory relief of pain and all 4 had had a revision from a previous arthroplasty.

Table 4

Pre- and post-operative pain assessment.

| PAIN | PRE-OPERATIVE | | POST-OPERATIVE | |
|---|---|---|---|---|
| None | 0 | ( 0% ) | 103 | (82%) |
| Mild | 0 | ( 0% ) | 19 | (15%) |
| Moderate | 0 | ( 0% ) | 3 | ( 2%) |
| Severe | 126 | (100%) | 1 | ( 1%) |

Although two thirds of the patients had rheumatoid arthritis with multiple joint involvement, 98% had a functional improvement following surgery. Seventy-seven per cent were able to walk more than 50 metres following surgery, compared with only 45% pre-operatively (Table 5).

Table 5

Pre- and post-operative mobility.

| MOBILITY | PRE-OPERATIVE | | POST-OPERATIVE | |
|---|---|---|---|---|
| Chairfast | 6 | ( 5%) | 0 | ( 0%) |
| Indoors only | 24 | (19%) | 11 | ( 9%) |
| <50m | 39 | (31%) | 17 | (14%) |
| >50m  < 500m | 45 | (35%) | 37 | (29%) |
| >500m <  1Km | 11 | ( 9%) | 38 | (30%) |
| >1Km | 1 | ( 1%) | 23 | (18%) |

The average pre-operative range of movement was 79° and the average fixed flexion deformity was 15°. Following surgery, the average range of movement increased to 96° and the average fixed flexion deformity was 3°. Two knees achieved 120° of flexion following surgery but 4 knees (3·2%) had less than 60°.

All knees except one were stable following surgery and the post-operative alignment as measured from weight-bearing radiographs showed 111 knees to be in valgus (range 1° - 14°, average 7°), 9 knees in varus (range 1° - 5°, average 4°) and 6 knees in neutral (this included the one unstable knee).

DISCUSSION

The aim of any joint replacement should be to achieve a painfree joint, with an active range of movement allowing normal function in an anatomical alignment, but it should not compromise bone stock. Earlier generations of knee arthroplasty have had problems with loosening of components (Watson and Hill 1976, Hui and Fitzgerald 1980, Matthews et al. 1986) and extensive loss of bone (Simison et al. 1986) thus making exchange arthroplasty difficult because of inadequate bony support. Following their removal a poor surface for an arthrodesis of the knee was left (Broderson et al. 1979, Fahmy et al. 1984).

Many of the patients in our series had rheumatoid arthritis and demonstrated severe pre-operative deformities with gross instability, but with adequate soft tissue release and correct alignment of the implant excellent early results have been achieved. We see little future for hinged or linked prostheses.

The relatively high overall complication rate demonstrated the rather poor general health of many of the patients. Many of the patients with rheumatoid arthritis had been on high doses of steroid therapy for several years.

The incidence of anterior knee pain following arthroplasty has been reported to be as high as 50% without resurfacing of the patella, (Mochizuki and Schurman 1979, Scott 1979, Clayton and Thirupathi 1982, Soudry et al. 1986), but in our series, when the patella was routinely resurfaced, anterior knee pain has not been a problem.

## CONCLUSION

The results in this series compare favourably with those described by Insall and co-authors (1979). The procedure is relatively simple and versatile, it conserves bone stock and is proving to be a reliable and robust prosthesis.

## REFERENCES

Broderson, M. P., Fitzgerald, R. H., Peterson, L. F., Coventry, M. B. and Bryan, R. S. (1979). Arthrodesis of the knee following failed total knee arthroplasty. Journal of Bone and Joint Surgery, 61-A: 181-185.

Clayton, M. L. and Thirupathi, R. (1982). Patellar complications after total condylar arthroplasty. Clinical Orthopaedics and Related Research, 170: 152-155.

Fahmy, N. R. M., Barnes, K. L. and Noble, J. (1984). A technique for difficult arthrodesis of the knee. Journal of Bone and Joint Surgery, 66-B: 367-370.

Fox, J. L. and Poss, R. (1981). The role of manipulation following total knee replacement. Journal of Bone and Joint Surgery, 63-A:

357-362.

Hui, F. C. and Fitzgerald, R. H. (1980). Hinged total knee arthroplasty. Journal of Bone and Joint Surgery, 62-A: 513-519.

Insall, J., Scott, N. and Ranawat, C. S. (1979). The total condylar knee prosthesis. Journal of Bone and Joint Surgery, 61-A: 173-180.

Insall, J. and Kelly, M. (1986). The total condylar prosthesis. A report of 220 cases. Clinical Orthopaedics and Related Research, 205: 43-48.

Matthews, L. S., Goldstein, S. A., Kolowich, P. A. and Kaufer, H. (1986). Spherocentric arthroplasty of the knee. A long-term and final follow-up evaluation. Clinical Orthopaedics and Related Research, 205: 58-66.

Mochizuki, R. M. and Schurman, D. J. (1979). Patellar complications following total knee arthroplasty. Journal of Bone and Joint Surgery, 61-A: 879-883.

Scott, R. D. (1979). Prosthetic replacement of the patello-femoral joint. Orthopaedic Clinics of North America, 10: 129-137.

Scott, R. D. and Volatile, T. B. (1986). Twelve years' experience with posterior cruciate-retaining total knee arthroplasty. Clinical Orthopaedics and Related Research, 205: 100-107.

Simison, A. J. M., Noble, J. and Hardinge, K. (1986). Complications of the Attenborough knee replacement. Journal of Bone and Joint Surgery, 68-B: 100-105.

Soudry, M., Mestriner, L. A., Binazzi, R. and Insall, J. N. (1986). Total knee arthroplasty without patella resurfacing. Clinical Orthopaedics and Related Research, 205: 166-170.

Watson, J. R. and Hill, R. C. J. (1976). The Shiers arthroplasty of the knee. Journal of Bone and Joint Surgery, 58-B: 300-304.

# 44

# CARBON FIBRE ARTHROPLASTY OF THE KNEE:  PRELIMINARY CLINICAL  EXPERIENCE IN A NEW CONCEPT OF BIOLOGICAL RESURFACING

R. J. Minns
J. A. Betts
D. S. Muckle
P. L. Frank
D. I. Walker
A. Strover
K. Hardinge

## INTRODUCTION

The  repair  of grade II articular cartilage defects (that is erosion of articular cartilage down to subchondral bone) in the knee  by  articular surface  drilling  to  achieve a fibrocartilage surface from subchondral bone has had only a limited  success.    Drilling  alone  may  encourage vascularization  and a fibrous response in small defects less than 1 cm. in diameter, but the repair of larger grade II defects by  chondrectomy and drilling has been particularly disappointing.

We  were intrigued by the intense organized fibrous response, seen in animals and humans, to carbon  fibre  for  ligament  reconstruction  and considered  applying  the  features  of  this  response  in a controlled fashion for the repair of grade II articular cartilage  defects  in  the knee.    The  material  has  many  attractions.    In its pure form it is chemically inert, is biocompatible in the environment of  the  knee  and induces  an  abundant  collagenous  fibrous  tissue organized around and along the carbon fibres.

## MATERIALS, METHODS AND PATIENTS

### Prosthesis design

Two designs  for  the  prosthesis  were  considered,  depending  on  the geometrical  and  physical conditions that the implants may be subjected to in the knee.   The first was a loosely woven pad of pure  filamentous carbon  fibre (fibre diameter of 9 micrometres) produced by conventional textile methods into pads of varying diameters of 8 to  32  mm.  and  a uniform  thickness  of  3 mm.   The open network of the weave produced a structure with over 85% porosity (or 15% carbon fibre volume). These pads were intended for use primarily on flat and concave surfaces in the knee. The second design was a braided rod, 3 mm. in diameter and 12·5 mm. long, the outer carbon fibres being braided to prevent disintegration of the central core of parallel aligned carbon fibres. The porosity of these rods was 50% by volume and they were placed in pre-drilled holes of a controlled depth on convex weight-bearing surfaces.

## Animal studies

Samples of woven carbon fibre pads 4 mm. diameter and 3 mm. thick were implanted into pre-drilled holes of 3 mm. depth in the weight-bearing area of the femoral condyles of adult New Zealand white rabbits, the contralateral femoral condyle in the other knee had an identical hole made with no implant.

Small samples of carbon fibre rods of 1 mm. diameter were implanted into another series of rabbits in a similar site and comparable observations were made.

## Surgical technique

### Pads

In areas of cartilage damage showing erosion down to subchondral bone in which the surface was flat or concave, the implants used were circular carbon fibre pads with diameters ranging from 8 to 32 mm. The subchondral bone was excised to a depth of approximately 3 mm. within the defect forming an undercut rim of 1-2 mm. The base usually was very well vascularized after preparing the implant site in this way. An appropriate sized pad of carbon fibre was pushed into the recess and fixed by squeezing into the undercut periphery.

### Rods

In areas of erosion needing carbon fibre rods of 3 mm. diameter, holes were drilled to a depth of at least 12 mm. controlled by a stop on the drill shank. The spacing recommended between rods was 1 cm. The top of the hole was enlarged by 1 mm. to accept a small cannula/introducer which was tapped into the enlarged end of the hole. The carbon fibre rod was introduced into the cannula top and a plunger of fixed length was used to push the rod into the hole in the subchondral bone to ensure that the rod end was either flush or below the articular surface.


## RESULTS

### Animal Studies

Histologically, the control hole from 4 weeks to 28 weeks had a similar appearance with a thin veil of fibrous tissue filling the outline of the hole boundary. In contrast from 4 weeks, the hole containing the implant was filled with a dense organized matrix of collagen-based fibrous tissue which invaded the trabeculae of the underlying subchondral bone. There was a pseudo surface of fibrocartilage covering the area. Fragmentation of the carbon fibres was not seen, as confirmed by scanning electron microscopy, even though the animals were allowed freedom of movement and presumably were weight-bearing on the implant site.

The main distinction seen with the implanted rods was the organizational feature of the fibrous tissue. The fibroblasts and collagen fibres appeared to align parallel to the axis of the rod in great abundance and emerge at the articular surface to form a "blister" of dense fibrous tissue over and surround the rod end. Tissue typing of the resulting fibrous material showed it to be all type 1, granulation collagen. The lateral surface of the hole showed invasion of this fibrous tissue into the bony trabeculae. In both designs of implant the foreign body reaction was very small with the presence of very few inflammatory cells around the individual carbon fibres. The results of these experiments are reported in full elsewhere (Minns et al. 1982).


### Clinical results

One hundred and forty-five knees in 138 patients have undergone carbon fibre arthroplasty in 2 of the collaborating centres; 79 males and 59 females with a mean age of 39 years and a range of 16 to 64 years. The decision to implant these prostheses was made at arthrotomy, most following arthroscopic diagnosis of the existence of grade II articular cartilage defects.

The dominant location of the carbon fibre pads was the patella ( 86 knees out of 93 ) and most of these pads were implanted on the medial and/or lateral facets (Figure 1 ).

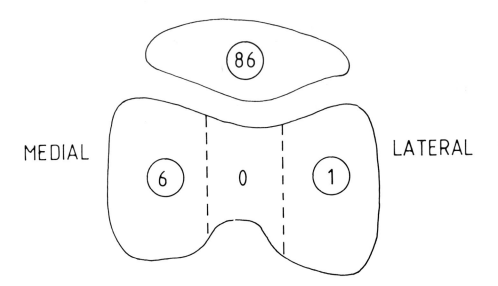

FIG. 1.  Location of pads in 93 knees.

In the case of the rods, 42 out of 118 knees rods were implanted into the patella, and a very similar number of knees had rods on the medial femoral condyle.  There were 18 knees with implants in the intercondylar and patellar groove areas and 17 knees and implants in the lateral femoral condyle (Figure 2).  The average number of rods in a knee was 5 with a range of 1 to 25.  Many cases in which a pad was inserted into the patella had rods implanted into a mirror lesion on the patellar groove (35 knees).

Subjective and clinical assessments were made 6 months to 5 years after carbon fibre arthroplasty and the results of these are shown in Table I.  Many of the patients demonstrated an excellent result and a return to function with a pain-free range of motion very quickly after surgery.

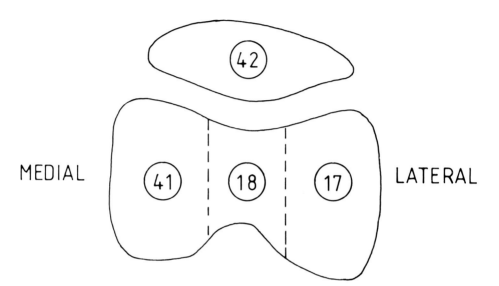

FIG. 2.    Location of rods in 118 knees.

TABLE I

SUBJECTIVE ASSESSMENT

145 KNEES

| | |
|---|---|
| ENTHUSIASTIC | 101 |
| SATISFIED | 31 |
| NON—COMMITTAL | 8 |
| POOR | 5 |

CLINICAL ASSESSMENT

| | |
|---|---|
| EXCELLENT | 108 |
| GOOD | 21 |
| FAIR | 11 |
| POOR | 5 |

Monitoring techniques have included follow-up arthroscopy 2 to 12 months after surgery in 75 patients and very few rods or pads were still visible after only 2 months of implantation. Blisters of fibrous tissue similar to those seen in the animal experiments were seen over the rod ends in areas which previously had been denuded of articular cartilage.

Four specimens have been retrieved by either implant removal because of continuing pain (2) or death (2). A whole patella containing a 20 mm. diameter carbon fibre pad was examined histologically and in the scanning electron microscope (Figure 3) to confirm that no fragmentation

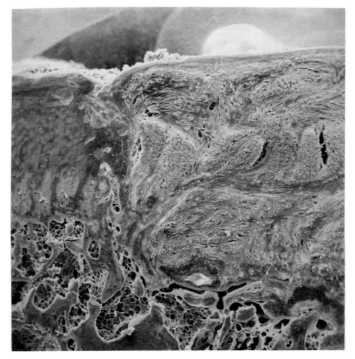

FIG. 3.    Scanning electron micrograph of the edge of the implanted carbon fibre pad (right), adjacent articular cartilage (left) and bone (bottom).

of the pad had occurred. Abundant fibrous tissue was seen to invade the implant interstices and the trabeculae of the subchondral bone, and this was covered by a thick (1 mm.) pseudo fibrocartilagenous surface, with similar features to that observed in the animal experiments. In the other 3 specimens, which were all carbon fibre rods, the fibrous material was abundant and protruded over the rod ends with good fibrous incorporation into the surrounding bone.


## DISCUSSION AND CONCLUSIONS

Carbon fibre is extremely strong in tension but has little strength in shear and bending and has virtually no "knotting" strength. As a consequence these implants should be positioned to avoid loading that would tend to cause fragmentation, i.e. the rods should be flush or below the articular surface, and the pads should not protrude outside the line of the original articular surface. When filled with fibrous tissue the resultant composite appears mechanically compliant and because of its viscoelasticity protects the carbon fibres from mechanical insult that would lead to fragmentation. In the 145 knees reported in this paper we have seen no evidence of disintegration in any of the pads or rods or of migration of carbon fibre debris into the joint space or surrounding tissues. An example of the decrease in load-bearing area capability of a lesion 20 x 60 mm. repaired with carbon fibre rods of 3 mm. at a spacing of 10 mm. is shown in Figure 4. In this example the reduction of area is only 4·6%: 95% of the subchondral bone is still able to bear load whilst the repair process is taking place.

Carbon fibre implants in the form of pads or rods placed in defects within the knee elicit a dense, organized matrix of fibrous tissue that forms a new biological and functioning articular surface. No evidence of implant fragmentation has been seen up to 5 years after implantation in the 145 knees studied. Carbon fibre arthroplasty appears to be appropriate in the surgical management of grade II articular cartilage lesions in the painful knee.


## REFERENCE

Minns, R. J., Muckle, D. S. and Donkin, J. E. (1982). The repair of osteochondral defects in osteoarthritic rabbit knees by the use of carbon fibre. Biomaterials, 3: 81-86.

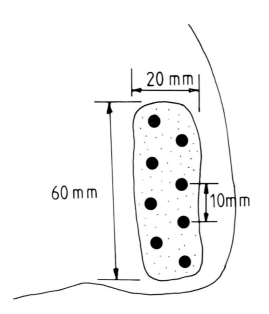

In a typical lesion measuring 20 × 60 mm, 8 rods used at a pitch of 10 mm

Carbon-fibre rods: dia.= 3mm, area = 7mm$^2$

Area of lesion = 20 × 60 = 1200 mm$^2$

Total area of rods used = 8 × 7 = 56 mm$^2$

∴ Ratio rods/total area = 56/1200

= 4·6 %

(Or remaining load bearing area 95·4% of original area of lesion )

FIG. 4.   The remaining load-bearing area after inserting carbon fibre rods 3 mm. in diameter and 10 mm. apart in a lesion 20 mm. x 60 mm.

## 45. VIBRATION ARTHROGRAPHY IN KNEE JOINT DIAGNOSIS

G. F. McCoy
D. E. Beverland
S. N. Shaw
W. G. Kernohan
R. A. B. Mollan

## INTRODUCTION

The detection and recording of vibration signals from human joints is a sensitive, non-invasive method for the objective study of the locomotor system. Attempts to correlate such signals with pathological lesions of the knee joint has a long history. In 1885, Heuter reported the first study involving the evaluation of sounds from the locomotor system when he described the localisation of loose bodies within the knee using a stethoscope. Since that time, many studies involving the evaluation of joint sounds have been reported. The earlier studies involved stethoscopic examination of the joints (Blodgette 1902, Bircher 1913, Walters 1929), but subsequently, to reduce subjectivity, microphones have been increasingly used (Erb 1933, Fischer and Johnston 1960, Danis et al. 1972). In 1974, Oehl and his colleagues used the term "phonoarthrography" to describe all microphone-based investigations of joint sounds. Despite the increasing sophistication of the computer recording and analysis techniques pioneered by Chu and others (1976a and b, 1978), microphone-based studies of joint sounds continued to be limited by the shortcomings of all acoustic systems: chiefly the poor response to low frequency signals and distortion caused by background noise.

The use of a vibration-sensitive sensor (or accelerometer) to record joint signals overcomes the problems inherent in acoustic systems. Mang, Birk and Blümel (1980) published the first such study using accelerometers. In doing so, they did not discuss their reasons for choosing accelerometers as sensors, nor did they appear to realise the significance of their choice. It was left to Mollan, McCullagh and Wilson (1982) and more recently to McCrea and colleagues (1985), working independently of Mang, to describe the considerable advantages of the use of vibration sensors to detect joint signals. Further work, reporting the application of vibration detection to other joints is now appearing in the literature (Cowie et al. 1984, Wallace et al. 1985). This paper reports our early experience of vibration detection in relation to the knee and discusses the clinical possibilities envisaged from further development of this technique. We propose that this technique be known as "vibration arthrography".


## MATERIALS, METHODS AND PATIENTS


The basic transducer used was a vibration sensitive device known as an accelerometer. This consisted of a piezo-electric crystal which responded to movement by producing a small voltage the size of which was directly proportional to the acceleration. The accelerometers were taped to skin preferably over bony prominences. Because they were sensitive to vibration at their point of application, the problem of background noise, which affected microphone-based systems, was minimised. Their small size and the fact that they could be securely fixed avoided skin friction noise. Cable distortion was removed by having pre-amplification with the accelerometer.

BBN Series 501 accelerometers of mass 1·8g, with integral pre-amplifiers, were chosen as the most suitable sensors. The output from the accelerometers was displayed in real time on an oscilloscope screen and was simultaneously recorded on a 4-channel FM tape recorder. The 4 channels allowed us to monitor the trace from 3 accelerometers attached around the knee while the fourth channel was used to record the signal from an electronic goniometer attached to the lateral aspect of the limb. The recording apparatus is seen attached to a subject in Figure 1.

For analysis purposes, each accelerometer output was fed in turn into a frequency analyser and, subsequently, into a microcomputer connected in series. In analysing each output channel individually, the maximal output channel and the relationship in size of signals to each other could be determined (McCrea et al. 1985). The signals were described using parameters which denoted the size of the "shock" (acceleration range), the power content (root mean square or RMS) and the peak frequency (Hz).

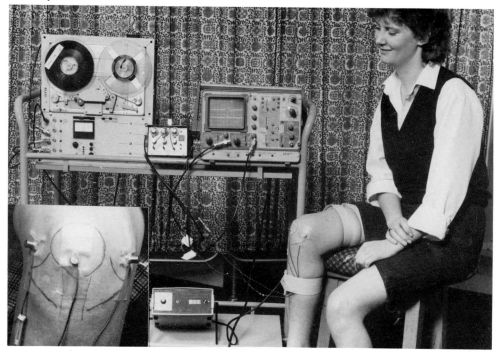

FIG. 1.   The  recording  equipment  attached to a subject with (inset)
standard positions of the accelerometers.

Using this method, we recorded and analysed the vibration output from
250 normal and 247 symptomatic individuals.   The normal subjects had no
past history of knee joint disorders, and  comprised  hospital  workers,
secondary  school  students  and  industrial  workers.   The symptomatic
patients had all been admitted for arthroscopy and underwent  a  testing
sequence  which  included  active  2,  4 and 6 second cycles, as well as
varus, valgus and McMurray stress cycles (a cycle being defined  as  one
complete  movement from 90° of flexion to full extension and back to 90°
flexion again).   A proportion of those patients who underwent  meniscal
excision  were re-submitted to vibration arthrography 3 months to 1 year
after surgery.


## RESULTS


One hundred and seventy-two of the 247 symptomatic subjects had meniscal
lesions  and  150 produced characteristic signals (diagnostic accuracy =

86%). The meniscal signal was quite unique and was produced by no other intra-articular pathology. A simultaneous displacement was observed on all 3 output channels with the maximal signal on the affected side. There were 85 cases of medial meniscus injury and 65 cases where the lateral meniscus was affected.

A variety of meniscal pathology was observed and the signal patterns recorded varied according to the meniscal lesion present. With a complete (Type I) bucket-handle tear, the signal characteristically occurred in mid-swing, close to 45°. With this type of lesion, the maximal displacement was seen over the patella with the smallest signal on the lateral side (Figure 2). With a type III lesion, occurring more towards the back of the joint, signals were observed at greater degrees of flexion (in the range 70-85°). The second largest displacement was seen over the opposite side, with the smallest signal over the patella. With a true posterior horn tear, the signal was recorded at 90° or greater, and the signal seen over the patella could be very small indeed.

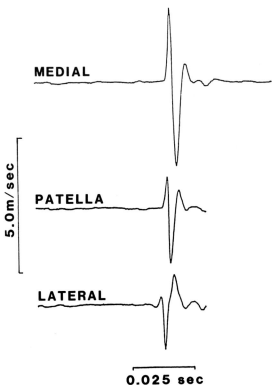

FIG. 2. Signal produced from a Type I bucket handle tear of the medial meniscus.

Surgery was found to have a profound effect on the meniscal signal. Twenty-six of the 150 signal producing patients, selected at random, were reviewed and recorded post-operatively. In 18 patients a resolution of the symptoms was accompanied by complete disappearance of the signal (Figure 3). In 5 patients minimal symptoms persisted and a much reduced signal was recorded post-operatively. In 3 patients the meniscal signal persisted undiminished in association with persistence of significant symptoms.

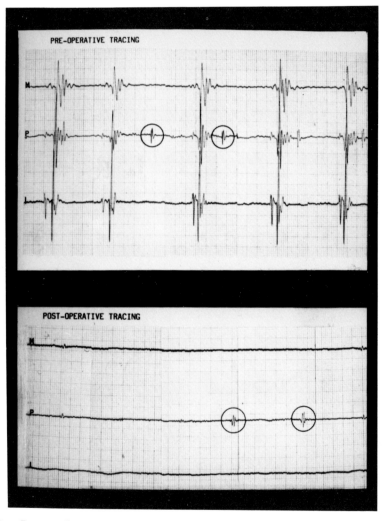

FIG. 3. Pre- and post-operative tracings of a patient with complete resolution of his symptoms. Note that the meniscal signal has completely disappeared, but a small "marker" signal (ringed) over the patella is seen in both tracings.

In all normal subjects when the knee was moved slowly a palpable patellar vibration was produced. It was only in advanced degenerative disease of the patellofemoral joint that this signal did not occur. We have called this signal "Physiological Patellofemoral Crepitus" (PPC). At angular velocities greater than 6° per second PPC was not produced.

## DISCUSSION

Our results, in respect of meniscal lesions, suggest that vibration arthrography is not only an accurate diagnostic technique, but also represents an objective method of assessment of the efficacy of arthroscopic meniscectomy.

It has been shown experimentally that PPC occurred as a result of slip-stick friction between the articular cartilage of the patella and the underlying trochlea. Many workers, such as Dowson (1967), have found that in vitro under static loads cartilage undergoes creep deformation. Concomitant with this deformation there was a rise in friction i.e. as cartilage deformed its coefficient of friction rose. We have been able to demonstrate this phenomenon **in vivo** by recording a baseline trace of PPC and then loading the knee isometrically for 10 seconds after which the signal was of a much larger amplitude.

The clinical implications of these findings are exciting but require evaluation. At one end of the spectrum a patient who had lost all articular cartilage due to degenerative disease produced no signal. At the other an individual with normal articular cartilage not only produced a signal but also exhibited an increase in amplitude of signal after isometric load as a result of cartilage deformation. Work is now continuing to control the production of PPC with the intention of being able to demonstrate quantitative/qualitative changes in PPC in conditions such as chondromalacia patellae.

## REFERENCES

Bircher, E. (1913). Zur Diagnose der Meniscusluxation und des Meniscusabrisses. Zentralblatt fur Chirurgie, 40: 1852-1853.

Blodgette, W. G. (1902). Auscultation of the knee joint. Boston Medical and Surgical Journal, 146:  63-66.

Chu, M. L., Gradisar, I. A., Railey, M. R. and Bowling, G. F. (1976a). An electroacoustical technique for the detection of knee joint noise. Medical Research Engineering, 12:  18-20.

Chu, M. L., Gradisar, I. A., Railey, M. R. and Bowling, G. F. (1976b). Detection of knee joint diseases using acoustical pattern recognition technique. Journal of Biomechanics, 9:  111-114.

Chu, M. L., Gradisar, I. A. and Zavodney, L. D. (1978). Possible clinical application of a non-invasive monitoring technique of cartilage damage in pathological knee joints. Journal of Clinical Engineering, 3: 19-27.

Cowie, G. H., Mollan, R. A. B., Kernohan, W. G. and Bogues, B. A. (1984). Vibration emission in detecting congenital dislocation of the hip. Orthopaedic Review, 13:  73-78.

Danis, L., Szabo, E. and Torok, Z. (1972). Genophonographiás á görbék osztályozása meniscus séruléseknél. Magyar Traumatologia, Orthopaedia Es Helyrequito Sebeszet, 15:  202-209.

Dowson, D., Longfield, M. D., Walker, P. S. and Wright, V. (1967). An investigation of the friction and lubrication in human joints. Proceedings of the Institution of Mechanical Engineering, 182:  68-76.

Erb, K. H. (1933). Uber die Moglichkeit der Registierung von Gelenkgeräuschen. Deutsche Zeitschrift fur Chirurgie, 241:  237-245.

Fischer, H. and Johnston, E. W. (1960). Analysis of sounds from normal and pathologic knee joints. In: Proceedings of Third International Congress - Physical Medicine, pp. 50-57.

Heuter, C. (1885). In: Grundriss der Chirurgie, Third Edition. (Ed. Vogel, F. C. W.), Leipzig.

Mang, W., Birk, M. and Blümel, G. (1980). Praktische anwendbarkeit der Phonoarthrographie in der Kniegelenksdiagnostik. Zeitschrift fur Orthopadie und Ihre Grenzgebiete, 118: 85-90.

McCrea, J. D., McCoy, G. F., Kernohan, W. G., McClelland, C. J. and Mollan, R. A. B. (1985). Vibrationsarthrographie in der Diagnostik von Kniegelenkskrankheiten. Zeitschrift fur Orthopadie und Ihre Grenzgebiete, 123: 18-22.

Mollan, R. A. B., McCullagh, G. C. and Wilson, R. I. (1982). A critical appraisal of auscultation of human joints. Clinical Orthopaedics and Related Research, 170: 231-237.

Oehl, R., Bohnenberger, J., Heinkelmann, W. and Petrowicz, O. Zur technik der phonoarthrogaphie. Medizinische Welt, 25: 1984-1989.

Wallace, R. G. H., Mollan, R. A. B. and Kernohan, W. G. (1985). Preliminary report on a new technique to aid diagnosis of some disorders found in hands. Journal of Hand Surgery, 10-B: 269-272.

Walters, C. F. (1929). The value of joint auscultation. Lancet, i: 920-921.

## 46.ROLE OF MAGNETIC RESONANCE IMAGING IN ORTHOPAEDICS

R. C. Mulholland

## INTRODUCTION

The phenomenon of magnetic resonance was discovered simultaneously by Bloch and Purcell in 1952, for which they were subsequently awarded the Nobel Prize. They discovered that atomic nuclei with an odd number of protons, when placed in a magnetic field and stimulated by radiowaves of specific frequencies, re-emitted some of the absorbed energy in the form of radiowaves. Different sequences of applied radiowaves produced different intensities of re-emitted radiowaves from different tissues. The use of gradient coils, each with a slightly different magnetic field, in three planes allowed spatial encoding of the signals and, hence, an image could be derived as each of these spinning nuclei sent a slightly different signal. If these signals were received by a receiver encircling the patient, the nuclear position and concentration could be recorded as an image.

As an imaging method the important features about magnetic resonance imaging (MRI) is its ability to image in any plane, its ability to differentiate tissues, and the fact that it does not involve the use of x-rays.

Most of our work has been in relation to the spine but, in many ways, the limbs are more suitable for MRI as they can easily be kept immobile during the examination. Furthermore, they are easily encircled by the receiver coils, achieving a better image as they are close to the tissue being imaged.

GENERAL MUSCULOSKELETAL IMAGING

This ability to image different tissues is illustrated in Figure 1
showing avascular necrosis of the femoral head.  The muscle layers are
clearly defined, and although cortical bone gives a poor image, the bone

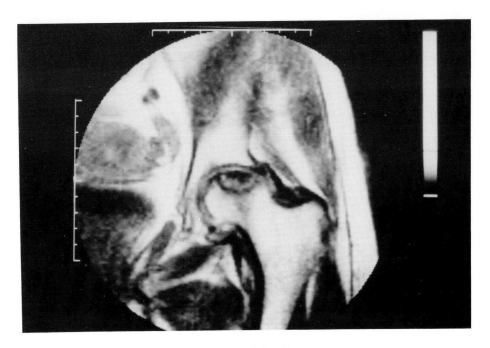

FIG. 1.  Avascular necrosis of femoral head.

is well outlined by the soft tissues.  The necrotic area is well shown.
Other joints can be imaged and, for example, in the knee the menisci are
well shown, as indeed are lesions of the meniscus, and collateral
ligament injuries.  A study by Reicher and others (1985) comparing
arthroscopy with MRI found an excellent correlation with no false
negative results for both cruciate and meniscal injuries.  Lesions of
the rotator cuff in the shoulder can also be demonstrated.

     The ability of MRI to discriminate between tissues and the
possibility of highlighting tissue differences by altered spin sequences
makes it of especial value in the assessment of soft tissue tumours
(Johnson in press).  In planning the surgical treatment of such tumours
information about the extent, other tissues involved, anatomical
position, and relation to major vessels is required.  MRI can provide
this as the muscles and vessels are well shown.  The investigation is

of particular value in the assessment of osteosarcoma.  Zimmer and
colleagues (1986) have demonstrated its superiority to CT in its ability
to demonstrate the soft tissue extent of the tumour, the spread in the
marrow, and especially the recognition of "skip lesion".  This is of
particular importance when evaluating the suitability of a tumour for
local resection, and prosthetic replacement.

Metastatic lesions in the bone, including spine, are well imaged.
This is of particular value in the spine, as relatively small
metastases, not apparent on plane films, will be shown.

Static blood produces a high signal, and fast flowing blood a very
low signal on MRI.  Hence, arteries and veins can be differentiated
and, indeed, a measure of blood flow can be made.  The vascular
potential of MRI has not been fully assessed; haematomata and other
soft tissue injuries can be imaged, as can venous thrombosis.  Vascular
anomalies, especially those in the spinal cord are well imaged.


SPINAL IMAGING


Disc disease
Our special interest in Nottingham was the application of MRI to the
spine and its value in the diagnosis of low back pain.

We have had particular experience in the use of discography as a
means of identifying disc degeneration as a source of single segment
instability, in the presence of normal radiographs, and confirming
normality of a disc above a proposed level of fusion.  Discography is a
painful, invasive procedure and because of the risk of infection,
potentially dangerous.  MRI clearly shows disc abnormality (Figure 2)
and to evaluate its accuracy we compared MRI with discography (Gibson et
al. 1986).  The results of the MRI and discography were reviewed
independently.  In 44 of the discs examined there was full agreement.
In the other 6, the failure of agreement was either due to observer
error in the interpretation of the discogram, or to misplacement of the
needle.  MRI has the great advantage that all the lumbar discs can be
imaged.  This is of particular importance as identification of the
symptomatic level in the lumbar spine is difficult, and a 5 level
discogram is a most invasive procedure.

MRI effectively images a disc protrusion in the sagittal plane;  less

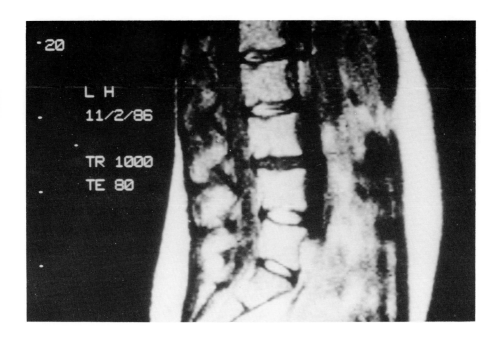

FIG. 2.  Degenerative L3/4 disc.

satisfactorily in the transverse plane.   However,  if  a  patient  with
clinical evidence of a protruding disc is imaged and a single level disc
abnormality is revealed, then that must be the level of the  protrusion,
as  in no case of surgically proven protrusion, that we have imaged, has
the MRI been normal.

The adolescent disc
We compared 20 asymptomatic adolescents with 14 adolescent patients with
myelographically  proven  disc  protrusions.   All  14 patients had MRI
abnormalities and 10 of the 14 had multiple level abnormality.   Only  4
of  the  asymptomatic  controls  had a disc abnormality.   These results
suggested that  disc  protrusion  not  only  occurred  in  a  previously
abnormal  disc, but since multiple level abnormality is usual, it really
represents  a  biochemical  failure,  probably  genetically  determined,
rather  than  primarily  a biomechanical failure.   A further suggestion
that mechanical failure is not the prime cause of disc  failure  is  the
fact  that  a number of patients with spondylolithesis have normal discs
on MRI.

## Value of MRI in spinal stenotic syndromes

One of the particular spin sequences that we have used was the so called
STIR sequence, the Short Tau Inversion Recovery sequence. This
produced an image of the spine which precisely reflected the image of
the lateral radiculogram, and could be used to assess canal stenosis, as
an alternative to the use of injected contrast. This may be of
particular value as, in these patients, there may be technical
difficulty in doing a radiculogram. Although CT gave a somewhat better
anatomical picture of the cortical bone and, therefore, delineates
precisely the subarticular region, MRI showed the soft tissue content of
the recess, particularly the fat content. This gives a very strong
signal which is lost in stenosis. In a couple of patients evaluated,
the CT scan provided excellent images showing subarticular stenosis
bilaterally where only one side was symptomatic, whereas the MRI image
revealed fat loss only on the symptomatic side. Loss of fat in the
intervertebral foramen was shown in the parasagittal plane in those
patients with canal stenosis. In a comparative study (Crawshaw et al.
1984) we found that MRI was as accurate as CT scanning in evaluating
lateral canal stenosis using the parasagittal plane.

## Value of MRI and Chymopapaine

We have had the opportunity to study the serial changes after injection
of Chymopapaine as we wished to establish whether clinical failure was
related to non-action of the enzyme. It clearly was not, as all
patients treated, whether clinically successful or not, developed marked
changes in the signal from the disc, analogous to premature disc
degeneration. What was of some surprise was that these changes,
presumably representing progressive biochemical alterations, in some
patients occurred over some months, rather than in the first few days as
might be expected from an enzymic response. A number of our
Chymopapaine treated patients have been followed for a couple of years
with serial MRI scans. There was no significant recovery of the
signal.

## Value of the STIR sequence in discitis and bone infection

Some of the Chymopapaine treated patients developed end-plate changes,
especially well shown on the STIR sequence. Most were transient but
this finding alerted us to the value of the STIR sequence in discitis.

We have subsequently found that MRI is a more sensitive examination than skeletal scintigraphy in the detection of disc infection, being positive at an earlier stage. Disc infection provided a very strong signal on the STIR sequence, distinguishing it from gross disc narrowing due to degeneration alone.

## DISCUSSION

What of the future? The Nottingham unit has a 0·15 Tessler magnet. The bigger magnets produce better images more quickly, whereas long imaging time with the smaller magnets is a significant problem, as some patients find the examination claustrophobic. With improved coils, further modification of spin sequences, and using somewhat bigger magnets, imaging quality and imaging time should markedly improve. Bigger magnets may allow the introduction into clinical use of soft tissue spectroscopy, allowing biochemical evaluation of altered physiology of tissues in disease. Patients are increasingly conscious about radiation, and such is the imaging potential and safety of MRI, that we must encourage development and assessment of MRI so that its role as an imaging technique can be established.

## ACKNOWLEDGEMENT

I would like to express my debt to Mr. C. Crawshaw, Mr. M. Gibson, and Mr. P. Szypryt, successive Spinal Research Fellows, who have done much of the work reported in this study.

## REFERENCES

Crawshaw, C., Worthington, B. S., Kean, D., Mulholland, R. S., Thomas, H. M., Preston, B. J., Hawkes, R. C., Moore, W. S. and Gyngell, M. (1984). The musculoskeletal application of NMR imaging. Journal of Bone and Joint Surgery, 66-B: 290.

Gibson, M. J., Buckley, J. H., Mawhinney, R. R., Mulholland, R. C. and

Worthington, B. S. (1986). A comparison of magnetic resonance imaging and discography in the assessment of intervertebral disc degeneration. A comparative study of 50 discs. Journal of Bone and Joint Surgery, 68-B: 369-373.

Johnson, R. J. (in press). Magnetic resonance imaging of musculo-skeletal sarcomata. In: Current Trends in Orthopaedic Surgery. (Eds. Galasko, C. S. B. and Noble, J.). Manchester University Press, Manchester.

Reicher, M. A., Rauschning, W., Gold, R. H., Bassett, L. W., Lufkin, R. B. and Glen W. (1985). High resolution magnetic resonance imaging of the knee joint. Normal anatomy. American Journal of Roentgenology, 145: 895-902.

Zimmer, W. D., Berquist, J. H., McLeod, R. A., Sim, F. H., Pritchard, D. J., Shives, T. C. and May, G. R. (1986). Magnetic resonance imaging of osteosarcomas. Comparison with computed tomography. Clinical Orthopaedics and Related Research, 208: 289-299.

## 47. AVASCULAR NECROSIS AND THE BLOOD SUPPLY OF THE FEMORAL HEAD

J. D. Spencer
M. Brookes

## INTRODUCTION

Avascular necrosis of bone (A.V.N.), ischaemic necrosis of bone, or osteonecrosis are some of the names given to a puzzling but crippling disorder of bone that affects steroid treated renal transplant patients. Because no definitive name for the condition could be agreed upon and because no two renal units had a similar incidence of A.V.N., we became interested, in 1978, to discover if further research could elucidate more information about this unusual complaint.

It was known that convex joint surfaces, most commonly the femoral head, were involved in steroid treated renal transplant patients. In some patients the lesions healed, in others gross destruction of bone occurred. Multiple joints might be involved, leading to severe disability in a young renal transplant patient. This lesion of bone appeared to lead to a subchondral fracture separating off normal articular cartilage and a layer of subchondral bone. The femoral head beneath exhibited a variable area of dead marrow and bone, and deep to this was highly vascular normal bone with granulation tissue. This lesion was seen in A.V.N. in patients with Caisson's disease, alcoholism, sickle cell disease, subcapital femoral fracture or hip dislocation, etc.

In the 1970's many investigators suggested theories as to the cause of steroid associated A.V.N. Fisher (1978) and Jones and co-authors (1965), following animal experiments with the administration of steroids in high dosage, thought that systemic fat embolism was produced, leading to occlusion of· small arteries in the femoral head. More recently, Ficat and Arlet (1980) suggested that idiopathic ischaemic necrosis of bone, which produced the same lesion as A.V.N., was caused by an

elevated intramedullary pressure, which obstructed venous drainage
inside the bone, leading to bone death.    Another recent theory (Kawai
et al. 1985) has diverted attention to intracellular fat deposition in
osteocytes.   This might lead to cell death and the production of A.V.N.

In the Guy's Hospital Renal Unit in 1978 it was evident that there
was an increase in the numbers of steroid treated renal transplant
patients developing A.V.N.    The first study (Spencer and Maisey 1985)
undertaken was designed to assess accurately the incidence of A.V.N.  in
renal transplant patients and to try to detect early the smallest
lesion.    Over 200 whole body bone scans were carried out in 42
consecutive renal transplant patients over a 2-3 year period using
Technetium labelled methylene diphosphonate (99m Tc-M.D.P.).    The scans
were carried out every 6 months and abnormalities confirmed by
radiographic examination, at operation or at post-mortem.     The
incidence of A.V.N. in these steroid treated renal transplant patients
using this method was 17%.    In one very early case a photon deficient
femoral head was seen on scintigraphy and because the patient died a few
weeks later, this femoral head was removed at post-mortem.
Histological examination of this and one other early case of A.V.N.
(both radiographically normal) showed small wedge shaped subchondral
infarcts of bone (Spencer et al. 1986).    This suggested that perhaps it
was the arterial blood supply of the femoral head that might be abnormal
in these patients.    In addition, no increase in fat cell size had been
seen in these 2 early cases and we were not able to confirm Ficat and
Arlet's finding of increased fat cell size in these patients.

This study was carried out to investigate the arterial and arteriolar
pattern of vessels in the femoral head of steroid treated renal
transplant patients, who during life were not known to have had any hip
joint disease.


PATIENTS AND METHODS


The study group consisted of 7 renal transplant patients on steroids and
Azathioprine and 3 dialysis patients who had never been on steroids.
The control group consisted of 6 patients who had died from myocardial
infarction, acute asthma, liver failure and breast carcinoma; but who
had not suffered from renal disease.

Warmed 45% micropaque was injected, usually via the common femoral artery at a constant pressure of 6 P.S.I., using a pump.  A volume of 2-4 litres of micropaque was used and a tourniquet applied around the lower thigh or knee.   The perfused femoral head was removed and immersed in a tank of buffered formal saline for 2 weeks before the bone was decalcified in 5% nitric acid.   The rectus femoris muscle was removed in all cases to check that the soft tissue had been adequately perfused.   All perfused femoral heads, from both the study and control groups, were cut into 4 mm. slices in the coronal plane after decalcification and microfocal radiography carried out on all available slices.   Histological 4 µm. sections were prepared from the central slice and stained with haemotoxylin and eosin.


## RESULTS


The femoral head arteriolar and arterial pattern was identical in the 3 dialysis and 5 of the 6 control patients.   The pattern of vessels in these cases was also identical with those obtained by Trueta and Harrison (1953).   The 2 renal transplant patients, who had died in the immediate post-operative period, were also shown to have a normal vascular pattern in the femoral head.

In the remaining 5 patients every single femoral head showed an abnormality of the arterial pattern.   Each patient had been asymptomatic as regards the hip joints, and they had been on steroids and Azathioprine for between 3 months and 4 years.   One patient was found to have multiple thrombi in the small arteries distal to one major, but not occluding thrombus in one of the lateral epiphyseal vessels (Figure 1).   In another patient an obvious area of subchondral bone without arterial or arteriolar vessels filled with micropaque could be seen (Figure 2).   New anastomotic channels were opening up around this dead area of bone.   Histological examination confirmed the presence of A.V.N. with dead osteones and marrow on an area larger than that suspected from the micropaque study.   This patient had no symptoms referrable to the hip joint or any other joint during life.

The 3 other steroid treated renal transplant patients had a paucity of micropaque filled vessels in the femoral head.   However, the adjacent soft tissues, periosteum and cortical bone of the neck of the

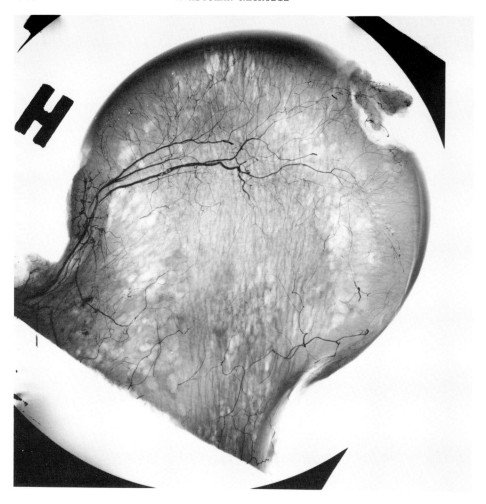

FIG. 1. Angiographic pattern of arteries in femoral head with multiple
filling defects (Patient T.H.).

femur had been perfused normally. In one of these patients, however,
the marrow sinusoids had excessively filled with micropaque, an
appearance similar to that produced by osteomedullography in patients
with early A.V.N. (Ficat and Arlet 1980).

   Histological examination showed that the smallest diameter of vessel
filled with micropaque was between 13–25 mm. Micropaque outlined the
femoral head and hip capsule vessels very clearly and microscopic
examination demonstrated arterial pathology in all 5 patients with
abnormal angiographic findings (Table 1). No abnormality of the
vessels was found in the 3 dialysis patients, the 2 renal
transplant patients who died in the immediate post-operative period, or

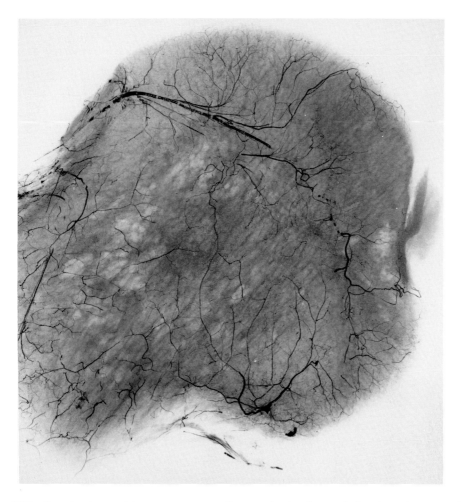

FIG. 2. Angiographic appearance of vessels in femoral head with area of necrosis of bone and bone marrow (Patient T.W.).

in any of the control patients. In addition, in the patient with multiple filling defects of the arteries of the femoral head, magnification of the radiographs showed very extensive longitudinal filling defects of many vessels in the femoral head. No other patient was found to have this abnormality.


## DISCUSSION


Although multiple theories have been advanced to explain the pathogenesis of A.V.N. in steroid treated renal transplant patients,

Table 1

Details of steroid treated renal transplant patients with   abnormalities
on micropaque injection study.

| Name | Angiographic pattern of vessels in femoral head | Histological abnormality of femoral head arteries | Thickening of capsular arteries on microscopy |
|------|-----|-----|-----|
| T.W. | Infarction | Degenerative Arterial Disease | +ve |
| T.H. | Filling defects in multiple arteries | Degenerative Arterial Disease | +ve |
| E.C. | Poor filling of arteries | None | +ve |
| D.C. | Poor filling of arteries | None | +ve |
| H.A. | Poor filling of arteries | None | +ve |

little research has been carried out in asymptomatic patients.   In this
study, 5 out of 7 asymptomatic patients were found to have abnormalities
in the  pattern  of arteries and arterioles in the femoral head.   This
was quite  unexpected  and  has  not  been  previously  described.   In
addition, histological examination revealed that degenerative changes in
the intima of arteries could occur in the capsule and  femoral  head  of
steroid  treated  renal  transplant  patients.   It is not inconceivable
that these abnormalities in the arteries of the femoral head and capsule
of  the hip joint found in asymptomatic renal transplant patients may be
related to the production of A.V.N.


REFERENCES

Ficat, R. P. and Arlet, J. (1980).   The  syndrome  of  bone  ischaemia.
In:   Ischaemia and Necroses of Bone.  (Ed. Hungerford, D. C.), Williams
and Wilkins, Baltimore, U.S.A., pp. 75–102.

Fisher, D. E. (1978).  The role of  fat  embolism  in  the  etiology  of
corticosteroid–induced  avascular  necrosis.   Clinical and experimental
results.  Clinical Orthopaedics and Related Research, 130:  68–80.

Jones, J. P., Engleman, E. P. and Najarian, J. S. (1965). Systemic fat embolism after renal homotransplantation and treatment with corticosteroids. New England Journal of Medicine, 273: 1453-1458.

Kawai, K., Tamaki, A. and Hirohata, K. (1985). Steroid induced accumulation of lipid in the osteocytes of the rabbit femoral head. A histochemical and electron microscopic study. Journal of Bone and Joint Surgery, 67-A: 755-763.

Spencer, J. D., Humphreys, S., Tighe, J. R. and Cumming, R. R. (1986). Early avascular necrosis of the femoral head. Report of a case and review of the literature. Journal of Bone and Joint Surgery, 68-B: 414-417.

Spencer, J. D. and Maisey, M. (1985). A prospective scintigraphic study of avascular necrosis of bone in renal transplant patients. Clinical Orthopaedics and Related Research, 194: 125-135.

Trueta, J. and Harrison, M. H. M. (1953). The normal vascular anatomy of the femoral head in adult man. Journal of Bone and Joint Surgery, 35-B: 442-461.